PLANT BASED COOKBOOK 2022

QUICK AND HEALTHY RECIPES FOR BUSY PEOPLE

JOE BROWN

Copyright 2022

All Rights Reserved

All rights reserved. No part of this book may be reproduced or copied in any form or by any means, electronic or mechanical, including photocopying, recording or by any information storage and retrieval system, without written permission from the publisher, except for the inclusion of brief quotations in a review.

Warning-Disclaimer

The aim of the information in this book is to be as accurate as possible. The author and publisher shall have neither liability or responsibility to anyone with respect to any loss or damage caused, or alleged to be caused, directly or indirectly by the information provided in this book.

Table of Contents

Introduction 10

Spiced Cauliflower Bites 13

Swiss-Style Potato Cake (Rösti) 15

Creamed Vegan "Tuna" Salad 17

Traditional Hanukkah Latkes 19

Thanksgiving Herb Gravy 21

Grandma's Cornichon Relish 23

Apple and Cranberry Chutney 25

Homemade Apple Butter 27

Homemade Peanut Butter 29

Roasted Pepper Spread 31

Classic Vegan Butter 34

Mediterranean-Style Zucchini Pancakes 35

Traditional Norwegian Flatbread (Lefse) 37

Basic Cashew Butter 39

Apple and Almond Butter Balls 40

Raw Mixed Berry Jam 42

Basic Homemade Tahini 44

Homemade Vegetable Stock 46

10-Minute Basic Caramel 49

Nutty Chocolate Fudge Spread 50

Cashew Cream Cheese 52

Homemade Chocolate Milk 54

Traditional Korean Buchimgae 55

Easy Homemade Nutella 57

Delicious Lemon Butter 59

Mom's Blueberry Jam 61

Authentic Spanish Tortilla 63

Traditional Belarusian Draniki 65

Mediterranean Tomato Gravy 68

Pepper and Cucumber Relish 70

Homemade Almond Butter 72

Indian-Style Mango Chutney 74

Easy Vegetable Pajeon 76

Healthy Chocolate Peanut Butter 78

Chocolate Walnut Spread 80

Pecan and Apricot Butter 82

Cinnamon Plum Preserves 84

Middle-Eastern Tahini Spread 85

Vegan Ricotta Cheese 87

Super Easy Almond Milk 89

Homemade Vegan Yogurt 91

South Asian Masala Paratha 94

Traditional Swedish Raggmunk 96

Buffalo Gravy with Beer 98

Spicy Cilantro and Mint Chutney 100

Cinnamon Almond Butter 102

Rainbow Vegetable Pancakes 104

Garden Tomato Relish 106

Crunchy Peanut Butter 109

Easy Orange Butter 111

Introduciton 114

LEGUMES 116

Traditional Indian Rajma Dal 117

Red Kidney Bean Salad 119

Anasazi Bean and Vegetable Stew 121

Easy and Hearty Shakshuka 123

Old-Fashioned Chili 125

Easy Red Lentil Salad 127

Mediterranean-Style Chickpea Salad 129

Traditional Tuscan Bean Stew (Ribollita) 132

Beluga Lentil and Vegetable Mélange 134

Mexican Chickpea Taco Bowls	136
Indian Dal Makhani	138
Mexican-Style Bean Bowl	140
Classic Italian Minestrone	142
Green Lentil Stew with Collard Greens	144
Chickpea Garden Vegetable Medley	146
Hot Bean Dipping Sauce	148
Chinese-Style Soybean Salad	150
Old-Fashioned Lentil and Vegetable Stew	153
Indian Chana Masala	155
Red Kidney Bean Pâté	157
Brown Lentil Bowl	159
Hot and Spicy Anasazi Bean Soup	161
Black-Eyed Pea Salad (Ñebbe)	163
Mom's Famous Chili	165
Creamed Chickpea Salad with Pine Nuts	167
Black Bean Buda Bowl	169
Middle Eastern Chickpea Stew	171
Lentil and Tomato Dip	173
Creamed Green Pea Salad	175
Middle Eastern Za'atar Hummus	178
Lentil Salad with Pine Nuts	180

Hot Anasazi Bean Salad 182

Traditional Mnazaleh Stew 184

Peppery Red Lentil Spread 186

Wok-Fried Spiced Snow Pea 188

Quick Everyday Chili 190

Creamed Black-Eyed Pea Salad 192

Chickpea Stuffed Avocados 194

Black Bean Soup 196

Beluga Lentil Salad with Herbs 200

Italian Bean Salad 203

White Bean Stuffed Tomatoes 205

Winter Black-Eyed Pea Soup 207

Red Kidney Bean Patties 209

Homemade Pea Burgers 211

Black Bean and Spinach Stew 213

Rainbow Chickpea Salad 216

Mediterranean-Style Lentil Salad 218

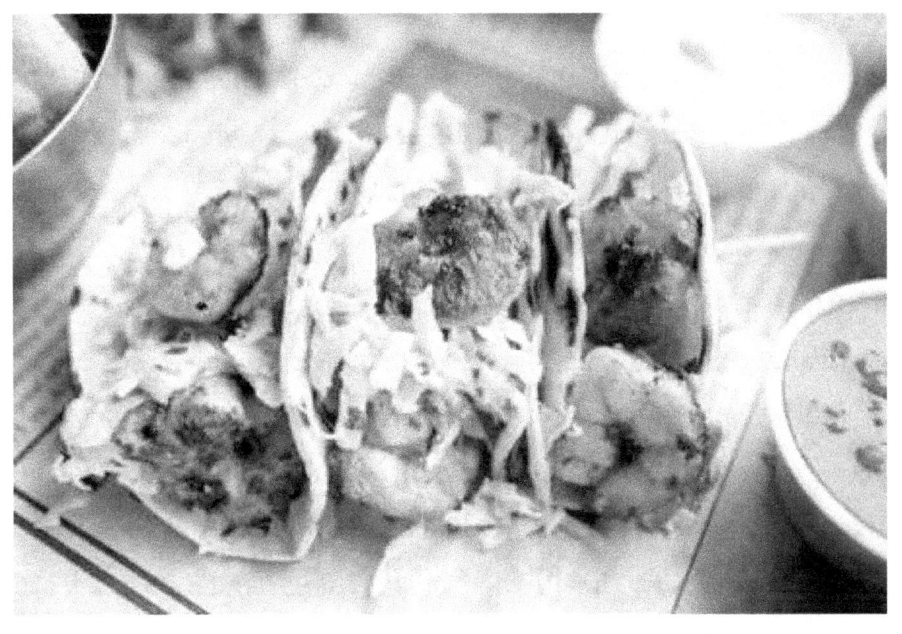

Introduction

It is only until recently that more and more people are starting to embrace the plant-based diet lifestyle. As to what exactly has drawn tens of millions of people into this lifestyle is debatable. However, there is growing evidence demonstrating that following a primarily plant-based diet lifestyle leads to better weight control and general health, free of many chronic diseases. What are the Health Benefits of a Plant-Based Diet? As it turns out, eating plant-based is one of the healthiest diets in the world. Healthy vegan diets include plenty of fresh products, whole grains, legumes, and healthy fats such as seeds and nuts. They are abundant with antioxidants, minerals, vitamins, and dietary fiber. Current scientific researches pointed out that higher consumption of plant-based foods is associated with a lower risk of mortality from conditions such as cardiovascular disease, type 2 diabetes, hypertension, and obesity. Vegan eating plans often rely heavily on healthy staples, avoiding animal products that are loaded with antibiotics, additives, and hormones. Plus, consuming a higher proportion of essential amino acids with animal protein can be damaging to human health. Since animal products contain much 8 more fat than plant-based foods, it's not a shocker that studies have shown that meat-eaters have nine times the obesity rate of vegans. This leads us to the next point, one of the greatest benefits of the vegan diet – weight loss. While many people choose to live a vegan life for ethical reasons, the diet itself can help you achieve your weight loss goals. If you're struggling to shift pounds, you may want to consider trying a plant-based diet. How exactly? As a vegan, you will reduce the number of high-calorie foods such as full-fat dairy products, fatty fish, pork and other cholesterol containing foods such as eggs. Try replacing such foods with high fiber and protein-rich alternatives that will keep you fuller longer. The key is focusing on nutrient-dense, clean and natural foods and avoid empty calories such as sugar, saturated fats, and highly processed foods. Here are a few tricks that help me maintain my weight on the vegan diet for years. I eat vegetables as a main course; I consume good fats in moderation – a good fat such as olive oil does not make you fat; I exercise regularly and cook at home. Enjoy!

Spiced Cauliflower Bites

(Ready in about 25 minutes | Servings 4)

Per serving : Calories: 187; Fat: 4.1g; Carbs: 32.8g; Protein: 6.2g

Ingredients

1 pound cauliflower florets

1 cup all-purpose flour

1 tablespoon olive oil

1 tablespoon tomato paste

1 teaspoon onion powder

1 teaspoon garlic powder

1 teaspoon smoked paprika

1/2 teaspoon dried oregano

1/2 teaspoon dried basil

1/4 cup hot sauce

Directions

Begin by preheating your oven to 450 degrees F. Pat the cauliflower florets dry using a kitchen towel.

Mix the remaining ingredients until well combined. Dip the cauliflower florets in the batter until well coated on all sides.

Place the cauliflower florets in a parchment-lined baking pan.

Roast for about 25 minutes or until cooked through. Bon appétit!

Swiss-Style Potato Cake (Rösti)

(Ready in about 25 minutes | Servings 5)

Per serving : Calories: 204; Fat: 11g; Carbs: 24.6g; Protein: 2.9g

Ingredients

1 ½ pounds russets potatoes, peeled, grated and squeezed

1 teaspoon coarse sea salt

1/2 teaspoon red pepper flakes, crushed

1/2 teaspoon freshly ground black pepper

4 tablespoons olive oil

Directions

Mix the grated potatoes, salt, red pepper and ground black pepper.

Heat the oil in a cast-iron skillet.

Drop handfuls of the potato mixture into the skillet.

Cook your potato cake over medium for about 10 minutes. Cover the potatoes and cook for another 10 minutes until the bottom of the potato cake is golden brown. Bon appétit!

Creamed Vegan "Tuna" Salad

(Ready in about 10 minutes | Servings 8)

Per serving : Calories: 252; Fat: 18.4g; Carbs: 17.1g; Protein: 5.5g

Ingredients

2 (15-ounce) cans chickpeas, rinsed

3/4 cup vegan mayonnaise

1 teaspoon brown mustard

1 small red onion, chopped

2 pickles, chopped

1 teaspoon capers, drained

1 tablespoon fresh parsley, chopped

1 tablespoon fresh coriander, chopped

Sea salt and ground black pepper, to taste

2 tablespoons sunflower seeds, roasted

Directions

Mix all the ingredients until everything is well incorporated.

Place your salad in the refrigerator until ready to serve.

Bon appétit!

Traditional Hanukkah Latkes

(Ready in about 30 minutes | Servings 6)

Per serving : Calories: 283; Fat: 18.4g; Carbs: 27.3g; Protein: 3.2g

Ingredients

1 ½ pounds potatoes, peeled, grated and drained

3 tablespoons green onions, sliced

1/3 cup all-purpose flour

1/2 teaspoon baking powder

1/2 teaspoon sea salt, preferably kala namak

1/4 teaspoon ground black pepper

1/2 olive oil

5 tablespoons applesauce

1 tablespoon fresh dill, roughly chopped

Directions

Thoroughly combine the grated potato, green onion, flour, baking powder, salt and black pepper.

Preheat the olive oil in a frying pan over a moderate heat.

Spoon 1/4 cup of potato mixture into the pan and cook your latkes until golden brown on both sides. Repeat with the remaining batter.

Serve with applesauce and fresh dill. Bon appétit!

Thanksgiving Herb Gravy

(Ready in about 20 minutes | Servings 6)

Per serving : Calories: 165; Fat: 1.6g; Carbs: 33.8g; Protein: 6.8g

Ingredients

3 cups vegetable broth

1 ½ cups brown rice, cooked

6 ounces Cremini mushrooms, chopped

1 teaspoon dried basil

1 teaspoon dried oregano

1/2 teaspoon dried rosemary

1/2 teaspoon dried thyme

1/2 teaspoon garlic, minced

1/4 cup unsweetened plain almond milk

Sea salt and freshly ground black pepper

Directions

Bring the vegetable broth to a boil over medium-high heat; add in the rice and mushrooms and reduce the heat to a simmer.

Let it simmer for about 12 minutes, until the mushrooms have softened. Remove from the heat.

Then, blend the mixture until creamy and uniform.

Add the remaining ingredients and heat your gravy over medium heat until everything is cooked through.

Serve with mashed potatoes or vegetables of choice. Bon appétit!

Grandma's Cornichon Relish

(Ready in about 15 minutes + chilling time | Servings 9)

Per serving : Calories: 45; Fat: 0g; Carbs: 10.2g; Protein: 0.3g

Ingredients

3 cups cornichon, finely chopped

1 cup white onion, finely chopped

1 teaspoon sea salt

1/3 cup distilled white vinegar

1/4 teaspoon mustard seeds

1/3 cup sugar

1 tablespoon arrowroot powder, dissolved in 1 tablespoon water

Directions

Place the cornichon, onion and salt in a sieve set over a bowl; drain for a few hours. Squeeze out as much liquid as possible.

Bring the vinegar, mustard seeds and sugar to a boil; add in the 1/3 teaspoon of the sea salt and let it boil until the sugar has dissolved.

Add in the cornichon-onion mixture and continue to simmer for 2 to 3 minutes more. Stir in the arrowroot powder mixture and continue to simmer for 1 to 2 minutes more.

Transfer the relish to a bowl and place, uncovered, in your refrigerator for about 2 hours. Bon appétit!

Apple and Cranberry Chutney

(Ready in about 1 hour | Servings 7)

Per serving : Calories: 208; Fat: 0.3g; Carbs: 53g; Protein: 0.6g

Ingredients

1 ½ pounds cooking apples, peeled, cored and diced

1/2 cup sweet onion, chopped

1/2 cup apple cider vinegar

1 large orange, freshly squeezed

1 cup brown sugar

1 teaspoon fennel seeds

1 tablespoon fresh ginger, peeled and grated

1 teaspoon sea salt

1/2 cup dried cranberries

Directions

In a saucepan, place the apples, sweet onion, vinegar, orange juice, brown sugar, fennel seeds, ginger and salt. Bring the mixture to a boil.

Immediately turn the heat to simmer; continue to simmer, stirring occasionally, for approximately 55 minutes, until most of the liquid has absorbed.

Set aside to cool and add in the dried cranberries. Store in your refrigerator for up to 2 weeks.

Bon appétit!

Homemade Apple Butter

(Ready in about 35 minutes | Servings 16)

Per serving : Calories: 106; Fat: 0.3g; Carbs: 27.3g; Protein: 0.4g

Ingredients

5 pounds apples, peeled, cored and diced

1 cup water

2/3 cup granulated brown sugar

1 tablespoon ground cinnamon

1 teaspoon ground cloves

1 tablespoon vanilla essence

A pinch of freshly grated nutmeg

A pinch of salt

Directions

Add the apples and water to a heavy-bottomed pot and cook for about 20 minutes.

Then, mash the cooked apples with a potato masher; stir the sugar, cinnamon, cloves, vanilla, nutmeg and salt into the mashed apples; stir to combine well.

Continue to simmer until the butter has thickened to your desired consistency.

Bon appétit!

Homemade Peanut Butter

(Ready in about 5 minutes | Servings 16)

Per serving : Calories: 144; Fat: 9.1g; Carbs: 10.6g; Protein: 6.9g

Ingredients

1 ½ cups peanuts, blanched

A pinch of coarse salt

1 tablespoons agave syrup

Directions

In your food processor or a high-speed blender, pulse the peanuts until ground. Then, process for 2 minutes more, scraping down the sides and bottom of the bowl.

Add in the salt and agave syrup.

Run your machine for another 2 minutes or until your butter is completely creamy and smooth.

Bon appétit!

Roasted Pepper Spread

(Ready in about 10 minutes | Servings 10)

Per serving : Calories: 111; Fat: 6.8g; Carbs: 10.8g; Protein: 4.4g

Ingredients

2 red bell peppers, roasted and seeded

1 jalapeno pepper, roasted and seeded

4 ounces sun-dried tomatoes in oil, drained

2/3 cup sunflower seeds

2 tablespoons onion, chopped

1 garlic clove

1 tablespoon Mediterranean herb mix

Sea salt and ground black pepper, to taste

1/2 teaspoon turmeric powder

1 teaspoon ground cumin

2 tablespoons tahini

Directions

Place all the ingredients in the bowl of your blender or food processor.

Process until creamy, uniform and smooth.

Store in an airtight container in your refrigerator for up to 2 weeks. Bon appétit!

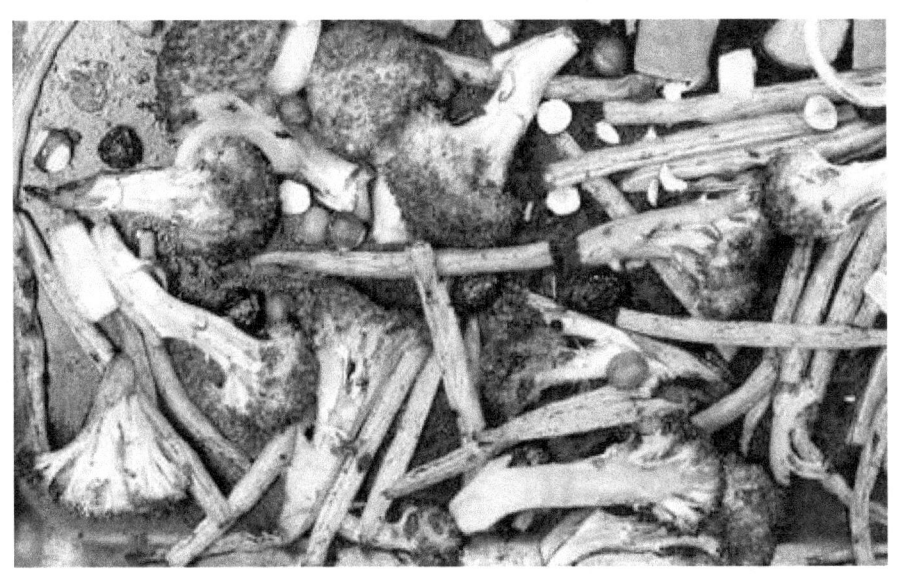

Classic Vegan Butter

(Ready in about 10 minutes | Servings 16)

Per serving : Calories: 89; Fat: 10.1g; Carbs: 0.2g; Protein: 0.1g

Ingredients

2/3 cup refined coconut oil, melted

1 tablespoon sunflower oil

1/4 cup soy milk

1/2 teaspoon malt vinegar

1/3 teaspoon coarse sea salt

Directions

Add the coconut oil, sunflower oil, milk and vinegar to the bowl of your blender. Blitz to combine well.

Add in the sea salt and continue to blend until creamy and smooth; refrigerate until set.

Bon appétit!

Mediterranean-Style Zucchini Pancakes

(Ready in about 20 minutes | Servings 4)

Per serving : Calories: 260; Fat: 14.1g; Carbs: 27.1g; Protein: 4.6g

Ingredients

1 cup all-purpose flour

1/2 teaspoon baking powder

1/2 teaspoon dried oregano

1/2 teaspoon dried basil

1/2 teaspoon dried rosemary

Sea salt and ground black pepper, to taste

1 ½ cups zucchini, grated

1 chia egg

1/2 cup rice milk

1 teaspoon garlic, minced

2 tablespoons scallions, sliced

4 tablespoons olive oil

Directions

Thoroughly combine the flour, baking powder and spices. In a separate bowl, combine the zucchini, chia egg, milk, garlic and scallions.

Add the zucchini mixture to the dry flour mixture; stir to combine well.

Then, heat the olive oil in a frying pan over a moderate flame. Cook your pancakes for 2 to 3 minutes per side until golden brown.

Bon appétit!

Traditional Norwegian Flatbread (Lefse)

(Ready in about 20 minutes | Servings 7)

Per serving : Calories: 215; Fat: 4.5g; Carbs: 38.3g; Protein: 5.6g

Ingredients

3 medium-sized potatoes

1/2 cup all-purpose flour

1/2 cup besan

Sea salt, to taste

1/4 teaspoon ground black pepper

1/2 teaspoon cayenne pepper

2 tablespoons olive oil

Directions

Boil the potatoes in a lightly salted water until they've softened.

Peel and mash the potatoes and then, add in the flour, besan and spices.

Divide the dough into 7 equal balls. Roll out each ball on a little floured work surface.

Heat the olive oil in a frying pan over medium-low heat and cook each flatbread for 2 to 3 minutes. Serve immediately.

Bon appétit!

Basic Cashew Butter

(Ready in about 20 minutes | Servings 12)

Per serving : Calories: 130; Fat: 10.1g; Carbs: 6.8g; Protein: 3.8g

Ingredients

3 cups raw cashew nuts

1 tablespoon coconut oil

Directions

In your food processor or a high-speed blender, pulse the cashew nuts until ground. Then, process them for 5 minutes more, scraping down the sides and bottom of the bowl.

Add in the coconut oil.

Run your machine for another 10 minutes or until your butter is completely creamy and smooth. Enjoy!

Apple and Almond Butter Balls

(Ready in about 15 minutes | Servings 12)

Per serving : Calories: 134; Fat: 2.4g; Carbs: 27.6g; Protein: 2.3g

Ingredients

1/2 cup almond butter

1 cup apple butter

1/3 cup almonds

1 cup fresh dates, pitted

1/2 teaspoon ground cinnamon

1/4 teaspoon ground cardamom

1/2 teaspoon almond extract

1/2 teaspoon rum extract

2 ½ cups old-fashioned oats

Directions

Place the almond butter, apple butter, almonds, dates and spices in the bowl of your blender or food processor.

Process the mixture until you get a thick paste.

Stir in the oats and pulse a few more times to blend well. Roll the mixture into balls and serve well-chilled.

Raw Mixed Berry Jam

(Ready in about 1 hour 5 minutes | Servings 10)

Per serving : Calories: 57; Fat: 1.6g; Carbs: 10.7g; Protein: 1.3g

Ingredients

1/4 pound fresh raspberries

1/4 pound fresh strawberries, hulled

1/4 pound fresh blackberries

2 tablespoons lemon juice, freshly squeezed

10 dates, pitted

3 tablespoons chia seeds

Directions

Puree all the ingredients in your blender or food processor.

Let it sit for about 1 hour, stirring periodically.

Store your jam in sterilized jars in your refrigerator for up to 4 days. Bon appétit!

Basic Homemade Tahini

(Ready in about 10 minutes | Servings 16)

Per serving : Calories: 135; Fat: 13.4g; Carbs: 2.2g; Protein: 3.6g

Ingredients

10 ounces sesame seeds, hulled

3 tablespoons canola oil

1/4 teaspoon kosher salt

Directions

Toast the sesame seeds in a nonstick skillet for about 4 minutes, stirring continuously. Cool the sesame seeds completely.

Transfer the sesame seeds to the bowl of your food processor. Process for about 1 minute.

Add in the oil and salt and process for a further 4 minutes, scraping down the bottom and sides of the bowl.

Store your tahini in the refrigerator for up to 1 month. Bon appétit!

Homemade Vegetable Stock

(Ready in about 55 minutes | Servings 6)

Per serving : Calories: 68; Fat: 4.4g; Carbs: 6.2g; Protein: 0.8g

Ingredients

2 tablespoons olive oil

1 cup onion, chopped

2 cup carrots, chopped

1 cup celery, chopped

4 cloves garlic, minced

2 sprigs rosemary, chopped

2 sprigs thyme, chopped

1 bay laurel

1 teaspoon mixed peppercorns

Sea salt, to taste

6 cups water

Directions

In a heavy-bottomed pot, heat the oil over medium-high heat. Now, sauté the vegetables for about 10 minutes, stirring periodically to ensure even cooking.

Add in the garlic and spices and continue sautéing for 1 minute or until aromatic.

Add in the water, turn the heat to a simmer and let it cook for a further 40 minutes.

Set a strainer over a big bowl and line it with cheesecloth. Pour the stock through and discard the solids.

Bon appétit!

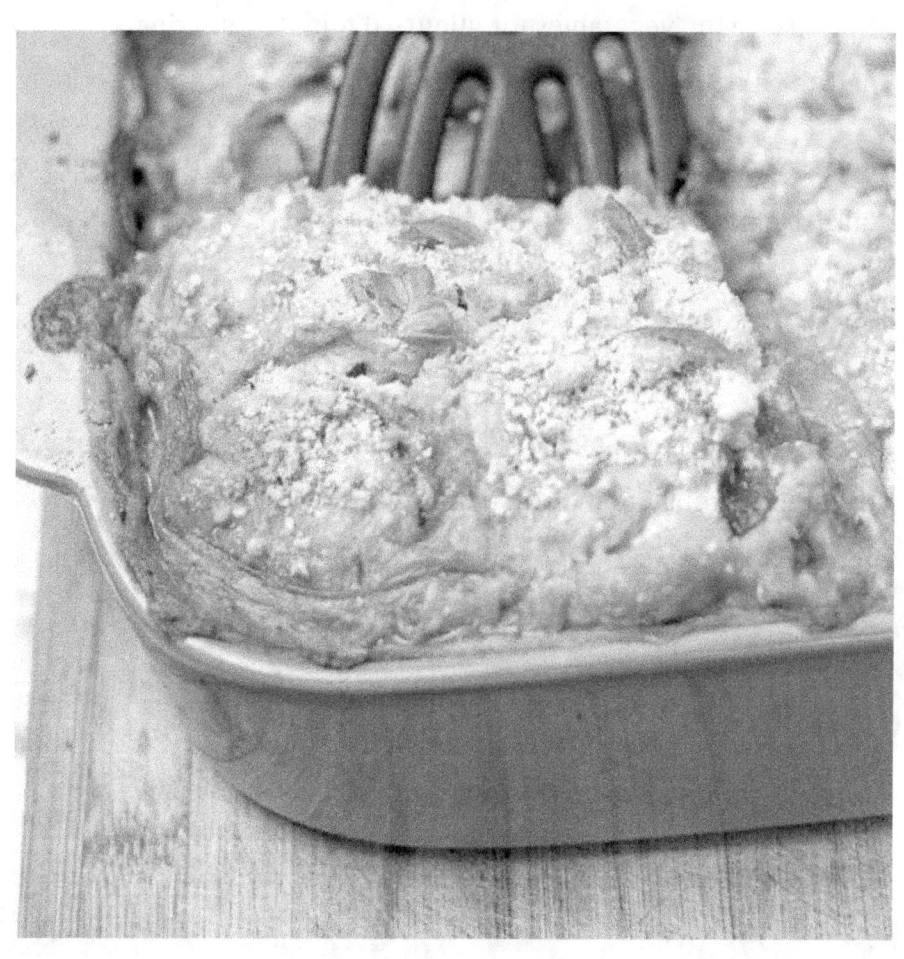

10-Minute Basic Caramel

(Ready in about 10 minutes | Servings 10)

Per serving : Calories: 183; Fat: 7.7g; Carbs: 30g; Protein: 0g

Ingredients

1/4 cup coconut oil

1 ½ cups granulated sugar

1/3 teaspoon coarse sea salt

1/3 cup water

2 tablespoons almond butter

Directions

Melt the coconut oil and sugar in a saucepan for 1 minute.

Whisk in the remaining ingredients and continue to cook until everything is fully incorporated and your caramel is deeply golden.

Bon appétit!

Nutty Chocolate Fudge Spread

(Ready in about 25 minutes | Servings 16)

Per serving : Calories: 207; Fat: 20.4g; Carbs: 5.4g; Protein: 4.6g

Ingredients

1 pound walnuts

1 ounce coconut oil, melted

2 tablespoons corn flour

4 tablespoons cocoa powder

A pinch of grated nutmeg

1/3 teaspoon ground cinnamon

A pinch of salt

Directions

Roast the walnuts in the preheated oven at 350 degrees F for approximately 10 minutes until your walnuts are fragrant and lightly browned.

In your food processor or a high-speed blender, pulse the walnuts until ground. Then, process them for 5 minutes more, scraping down the sides and bottom of the bowl; reserve.

Melt the coconut oil over medium heat. Add in the corn flour and continue to cook until the mixture starts to boil.

Turn the heat to a simmer, add in the cocoa powder, nutmeg, cinnamon and salt; continue to cook, stirring occasionally, for about 10 minutes.

Fold in the ground walnuts, stir to combine and store in a glass jar. Enjoy!

Cashew Cream Cheese

(Ready in about 10 minutes | Servings 6)

Per serving : Calories: 197; Fat: 14.4g; Carbs: 11.4g; Protein: 7.4g

Ingredients

1 ½ cups cashews, soaked overnight and drained

1/3 cup water

1/4 teaspoon coarse sea salt

1/4 teaspoon dried dill weed

1/4 teaspoon garlic powder

2 tablespoons nutritional yeast

2 probiotic capsules

Directions

Process the cashews and water in your blender until creamy and uniform.

Add in the salt, dill, garlic powder and nutritional yeast; continue to blend until everything is well incorporated.

Spoon the mixture into a sterilized glass jar. Add in the probiotic powder and combine with a wooden spoon (not metal!)

Cover the jar with a clean kitchen towel and let it stand on the kitchen counter to ferment for 24-48 hours.

Keep in your refrigerator for up to a week. Bon appétit!

Homemade Chocolate Milk

(Ready in about 10 minutes | Servings 4)

Per serving : Calories: 79; Fat: 3.1g; Carbs: 13.3g; Protein: 1.3g

Ingredients

4 teaspoons cashew butter

4 cups water

1/2 teaspoon vanilla paste

4 teaspoons cocoa powder

8 dates, pitted

Directions

Place all the ingredients in the bowl of your high-speed blender.

Process until creamy, uniform and smooth.

Keep in a glass bottle in your refrigerator for up to 4 days. Enjoy!

Traditional Korean Buchimgae

(Ready in about 20 minutes | Servings 4)

Per serving : Calories: 315; Fat: 19g; Carbs: 26.1g; Protein: 9.5g

Ingredients

1/2 cup all-purpose flour

1/2 cup chickpea flour

1/2 teaspoon baking powder

1 teaspoon garlic powder

1/4 teaspoon ground cumin

1/2 teaspoon sea salt

1 carrot, trimmed and grated

1 small onion, finely chopped

1 cup Kimchi

1 green chili, minced

1 flax egg

1 tablespoon bean paste

1 cup rice milk

4 tablespoons canola oil

Directions

Thoroughly combine the flour, baking powder and spices. In a separate bowl, combine the carrot, onion, Kimchi, green chili, flax egg, bean paste and rice milk.

Add the vegetable mixture to the dry flour mixture; stir to combine well.

Then, heat the oil in a frying pan over a moderate flame. Cook the Korean pancakes for 2 to 3 minutes per side until crispy.

Bon appétit!

Easy Homemade Nutella

(Ready in about 25 minutes | Servings 20)

Per serving : Calories: 187; Fat: 17.1g; Carbs: 7g; Protein: 4g

Ingredients

3 ½ cups hazelnuts

1 teaspoon vanilla seeds

A pinch of coarse sea salt

A pinch of grated nutmeg

1/2 teaspoon ground cinnamon

1/2 teaspoon ground cardamom

1 cup dark chocolate chips

Directions

Roast the hazelnuts in the preheated oven at 350 degrees F for approximately 13 minutes until your hazelnuts are fragrant and lightly browned.

In your food processor or a high-speed blender, pulse the hazelnuts until ground. Then, process the mixture for 5 minutes more, scraping down the sides and bottom of the bowl.

Add in the remaining ingredients.

Run your machine for a further 4 to 5 minutes or until the mixture is completely creamy and smooth. Enjoy!

Delicious Lemon Butter

(Ready in about 10 minutes | Servings 8)

Per serving : Calories: 87; Fat: 3.4g; Carbs: 14.6g; Protein: 0g

Ingredients

1/2 cup granulated sugar

2 tablespoons cornstarch

1/2 teaspoon lemon zest, grated

1 cup water

2 tablespoons fresh lemon juice

2 tablespoons coconut oil

Directions

In a saucepan, combine the sugar, cornstarch and lemon zest over a moderate heat.

Stir in the water and lemon juice and continue to cook until the mixture has thickened. Heat off.

Stir in the coconut oil. Bon appétit!

Mom's Blueberry Jam

(Ready in about 40 minutes | Servings 20)

Per serving : Calories: 108; Fat: 0.1g; Carbs: 27.6g; Protein: 0.2g

Ingredients

1 ½ pounds fresh blueberries

1 pound granulated sugar

1 cinnamon stick

5-6 cloves

1 vanilla pod, split lengthways

1 lemon, juiced

Directions

Mix all the ingredients in a saucepan.

Continue to cook over medium heat, stirring constantly, until the sauce has reduced and thickened for about 30 minutes.

Remove from the heat. Leave your jam to sit for 10 minutes. Ladle into sterilized jars and cover with the lids. Let it cool completely.

Bon appétit!

Authentic Spanish Tortilla

(Ready in about 30 minutes | Servings 4)

Per serving : Calories: 365; Fat: 13.9g; Carbs: 48.1g; Protein: 14.5g

Ingredients

2 tablespoons olive oil

1 ½ pounds russet potatoes, peeled and sliced

1 onion, chopped

Sea salt and ground black pepper, to taste

1/4 cup rice milk

8 ounces tofu, pressed and drained

1/2 cup besan

2 tablespoons cornstarch

1/2 teaspoon ground cumin

1/4 teaspoon ground allspice

Directions

Heat 1 tablespoon of the olive oil in a frying pan. Then, add the potatoes, onion, salt and black pepper to the frying pan.

Cook for about 20 minutes or until the potatoes have softened.

In a mixing bowl, thoroughly combine the remaining ingredients. Add in the potato mixture and stir to combine.

Heat the remaining 1 tablespoon of the olive oil in a frying pan over medium-low heat. Cook your tortilla for 5 minutes per side. Serve warm.

Bon appétit!

Traditional Belarusian Draniki

(Ready in about 30 minutes | Servings 4)

Per serving : Calories: 350; Fat: 14.4g; Carbs: 45.6g; Protein: 6.8g

Ingredients

4 waxy potatoes, peeled, grated and squeezed

4 tablespoons scallions, chopped

1 green chili pepper, chopped

1 red chili pepper, chopped

1/3 cup besan

1/2 teaspoon baking powder

1 teaspoon paprika

Sea salt and red pepper, to taste

1/4 cup canola oil

2 tablespoons fresh cilantro, chopped

Directions

Thoroughly combine the grated potatoes, scallions, pepper, besan, baking powder, paprika, salt and red pepper.

Preheat the oil in a frying pan over a moderate heat.

Spoon 1/4 cup of potato mixture into the pan and cook your draniki until golden brown on both sides. Repeat with the remaining batter.

Serve with fresh cilantro. Bon appétit!

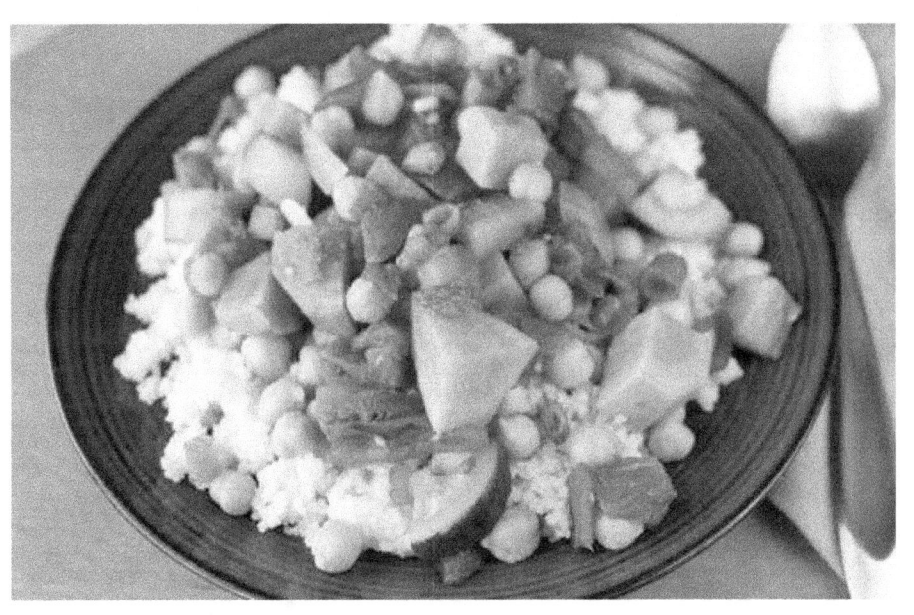

Mediterranean Tomato Gravy

(Ready in about 20 minutes | Servings 6)

Per serving : Calories: 106; Fat: 6.6g; Carbs: 9.6g; Protein: 0.8g

Ingredients

3 tablespoons olive oil

1 red onion, chopped

3 cloves garlic, crushed

4 tablespoons cornstarch

1 can (14 ½-ounce) tomatoes, crushed

1/2 teaspoon dried basil

1/2 teaspoon dried oregano

1/2 teaspoon dried thyme

1 teaspoon dried parsley flakes

Sea salt and black pepper, to taste

Directions

Heat the olive oil in a large saucepan over medium-high heat. Once hot, sauté the onion and garlic until tender and fragrant.

Add in the cornstarch and continue to cook for 1 minute more.

Add in the canned tomatoes and bring to a boil over medium-high heat; stir in the spices and turn the heat to a simmer.

Let it simmer for about 10 minutes until everything is cooked through.

Serve with vegetables of choice. Bon appétit!

Pepper and Cucumber Relish

(Ready in about 20 minutes + chilling time | Servings 10)

Per serving : Calories: 66; Fat: 0.3g; Carbs: 15.3g; Protein: 1.5g

Ingredients

6 cucumbers, chopped

1 red bell pepper, seeded and chopped

1 green bell pepper, seeded and chopped

2 tablespoons coarse sea salt

1/2 cup wine vinegar

2/3 cup granulated sugar

1/2 teaspoon fennel seeds

1/4 teaspoon mustard seeds

1/4 teaspoon ground turmeric

1/2 teaspoon ground allspice

1 tablespoon mixed peppercorns

4 teaspoons cornstarch

Directions

Place the cucumber, bell pepper and salt in a sieve set over a bowl; drain for a few hours. Squeeze out as much liquid as possible.

Bring the vinegar and sugar to a boil; add in the 1/3 teaspoon of the sea salt and let it boil until the sugar has dissolved.

Add in the cucumber-pepper mixture and continue to simmer for 2 to 3 minutes more. Stir in the spices and cornstarch; continue to simmer for 1 to 2 minutes more.

Transfer the relish to a bowl and place, uncovered, in your refrigerator for about 2 hours. Bon appétit!

Homemade Almond Butter

(Ready in about 20 minutes | Servings 20)

Per serving : Calories: 131; Fat: 11.3g; Carbs: 4.8g; Protein: 4.8g

Ingredients

1 pound almonds

A pinch of sea salt

A pinch of grated nutmeg

Directions

Roast the almonds in the preheated oven at 350 degrees F for approximately 9 minutes until your nuts are fragrant and lightly browned.

In your food processor or a high-speed blender, pulse the almonds until ground. Then, process the mixture for 5 minutes more, scraping down the sides and bottom of the bowl.

Add in the salt and nutmeg.

Run your machine for another 10 minutes or until your butter is completely creamy and smooth. Enjoy!

Indian-Style Mango Chutney

(Ready in about 1 hour | Servings 7)

Per serving : Calories: 273; Fat: 2.3g; Carbs: 64.3g; Protein: 2.4g

Ingredients

5 mangoes, peeled and diced

1 yellow onion, chopped

2 red chilies, chopped

3/4 cup balsamic vinegar

1 ½ cups granulated sugar

1 teaspoon coriander seeds

1 tablespoon chana dal

1/2 teaspoon jeera

1/4 teaspoon turmeric powder

1/4 teaspoon Himalayan salt

1/2 cup currants

Directions

In a saucepan, place the mangoes, onion, red chilies, vinegar, granulated sugar, coriander seeds, chana dal, jeera, turmeric powder and salt. Bring the mixture to a boil.

Immediately turn the heat to simmer; continue to simmer, stirring occasionally, for approximately 55 minutes, until most of the liquid has absorbed.

Set aside to cool and add in the currants. Store in your refrigerator for up to 2 weeks.

Bon appétit!

Easy Vegetable Pajeon

(Ready in about 20 minutes | Servings 4)

Per serving : Calories: 255; Fat: 10.6g; Carbs: 33.3g; Protein: 6.2g

Ingredients

1/2 cup all-purpose flour

1/2 cup potato starch

1 teaspoon baking powder

1/3 teaspoon Himalayan salt

1/2 cup kimchi, finely chopped

4 scallions, chopped

1 carrot, trimmed and chopped

2 bell peppers, chopped

1 green chili pepper, chopped

1 cup kimchi liquid

2 tablespoons olive oil

Dipping sauce:

2 tablespoons soy sauce

2 teaspoons rice vinegar

1 teaspoon fresh ginger, finely grated

Directions

Thoroughly combine the flour, potato starch, baking powder and salt. In a separate bowl, combine the vegetables and kimchi liquid.

Add the vegetable mixture to the dry flour mixture; stir to combine well.

Then, heat the oil in a frying pan over a moderate flame. Cook the Pajeon for 2 to 3 minutes per side until crispy.

Meanwhile, mix the sauce ingredients. Serve your Pajeon with the sauce for dipping. Bon appétit!

Healthy Chocolate Peanut Butter

(Ready in about 15 minutes | Servings 20)

Per serving : Calories: 118; Fat: 9.2g; Carbs: 6.9g; Protein: 5.1g

Ingredients

- 2 ½ cups peanuts
- 1/2 teaspoon coarse sea salt
- 1/2 teaspoon cinnamon powder
- 1/2 cup cocoa powder
- 10 dates, pitted

Directions

Roast the peanuts in the preheated oven at 350 degrees F for approximately 7 minutes until the peanuts are fragrant and lightly browned.

In your food processor or a high-speed blender, pulse the peanuts until ground. Then, process the mixture for 2 minutes more, scraping down the sides and bottom of the bowl.

Add in the salt, cinnamon, cocoa powder and dates.

Run your machine for another 2 minutes or until your butter is completely creamy and smooth. Enjoy!

Chocolate Walnut Spread

(Ready in about 20 minutes | Servings 15)

Per serving : Calories: 78; Fat: 4.7g; Carbs: 9g; Protein: 1.5g

Ingredients

1 cup walnuts

1 teaspoon pure vanilla extract

1/2 cup agave nectar

4 tablespoons cocoa powder

A pinch of ground cinnamon

A pinch of grated nutmeg

A pinch of sea salt

4 tablespoons almond milk

Directions

Roast the walnuts in the preheated oven at 350 degrees F for approximately 10 minutes until they are fragrant and lightly browned.

In your food processor or a high-speed blender, pulse the walnuts until ground. Then, process the mixture for 5 minutes more, scraping down the sides and bottom of the bowl.

Add in the remaining ingredients.

Run your machine for a further 5 minutes or until the mixture is completely creamy and smooth. Enjoy!

Pecan and Apricot Butter

(Ready in about 15 minutes | Servings 16)

Per serving : Calories: 163; Fat: 17g; Carbs: 2.5g; Protein: 1.4g

Ingredients

2 ½ cups pecans

1/2 cup dried apricots, chopped

1/2 cup sunflower oil

1 teaspoon bourbon vanilla

1/4 teaspoon ground anise

1/2 teaspoon cinnamon

1/8 teaspoon grated nutmeg

1/8 teaspoon salt

Directions

In your food processor or a high-speed blender, pulse the pecans until ground. Then, process the pecans for 5 minutes more, scraping down the sides and bottom of the bowl.

Add in the remaining ingredients.

Run your machine for a further 5 minutes or until the mixture is completely creamy and smooth. Enjoy!

Cinnamon Plum Preserves

(Ready in about 40 minutes | Servings 20)

Per serving : Calories: 223; Fat: 0.3g; Carbs: 58.1g; Protein: 0.8g

Ingredients

5 pounds ripe plums rinsed

2 pounds granulated sugar

2 tablespoons lemon juice

3 cinnamon sticks

Directions

Mix all the ingredients in a saucepan.

Continue to cook over medium heat, stirring constantly, until the sauce has reduced and thickened for about 30 minutes.

Remove from the heat. Leave your jam to sit for 10 minutes. Ladle into sterilized jars and cover with the lids. Let it cool completely.

Bon appétit!

Middle-Eastern Tahini Spread

(Ready in about 10 minutes | Servings 16)

Per serving : Calories: 143; Fat: 13.3g; Carbs: 6.2g; Protein: 3.9g

Ingredients

- 10 ounces sesame seeds
- 3 tablespoons cocoa powder
- 1 teaspoon vanilla seeds
- 1/4 teaspoon kosher salt
- 1/2 cup fresh dates, pitted
- 3 tablespoons coconut oil

Directions

Toast the sesame seeds in a nonstick skillet for about 4 minutes, stirring continuously. Cool the sesame seeds completely.

Transfer the sesame seeds to the bowl of your food processor. Process for about 1 minute.

Add in the remaining ingredients and process for a further 4 minutes, scraping down the bottom and sides of the bowl.

Store your tahini spread in the refrigerator for up to 1 month. Bon appétit!

Vegan Ricotta Cheese

(Ready in about 10 minutes | Servings 12)

Per serving : Calories: 74; Fat: 6.3g; Carbs: 3.3g; Protein: 2.7g

Ingredients

1/2 cup raw cashew nuts, soaked overnight and drained

1/2 cup raw sunflower seeds, soaked overnight and drained

1/4 cup water

1 heaping tablespoon coconut oil, melted

1 tablespoon lime juice, freshly squeezed

1 tablespoon white vinegar

1/4 teaspoon Dijon mustard

2 tablespoons nutritional yeast

1/2 teaspoon garlic powder

1/2 teaspoon turmeric powder

1/2 teaspoon salt

Directions

Process the cashews, sunflower seeds and water in your blender until creamy and uniform.

Add in the remaining ingredients; continue to blend until everything is well incorporated.

Keep in your refrigerator for up to a week. Bon appétit!

Super Easy Almond Milk

(Ready in about 10 minutes | Servings 6)

Per serving : Calories: 78; Fat: 6g; Carbs: 4.8g; Protein: 2.5g

Ingredients

1 cup raw almonds, soaked overnight and drained

6 cups water

1 tablespoon maple syrup

A pinch of grated nutmeg

A pinch of salt

A pinch of ground cinnamon

1 teaspoon vanilla extract

Directions

Place all the ingredients in the bowl of your high-speed blender.

Process until creamy, uniform and smooth.

Strain the liquid using a nut milk bag; squeeze until all of the liquid is extracted.

Keep in a glass bottle in your refrigerator for up to 4 days. Enjoy!

Homemade Vegan Yogurt

(Ready in about 10 minutes | Servings 6)

Per serving : Calories: 141; Fat: 14.2g; Carbs: 4g; Protein: 1.3g

Ingredients

1 ½ cups full-fat coconut milk

1 teaspoon maple syrup

A pinch of coarse sea salt

2 capsules vegan probiotic

Directions

Spoon the coconut milk into a sterilized glass jar. Add in the maple syrup and salt.

Empty your probiotic capsules and stir with a wooden spoon (not metal!)

Cover the jar with a clean kitchen towel and let it stand on the kitchen counter to ferment for 24-48 hours.

Keep in your refrigerator for up to a week. Bon appétit!

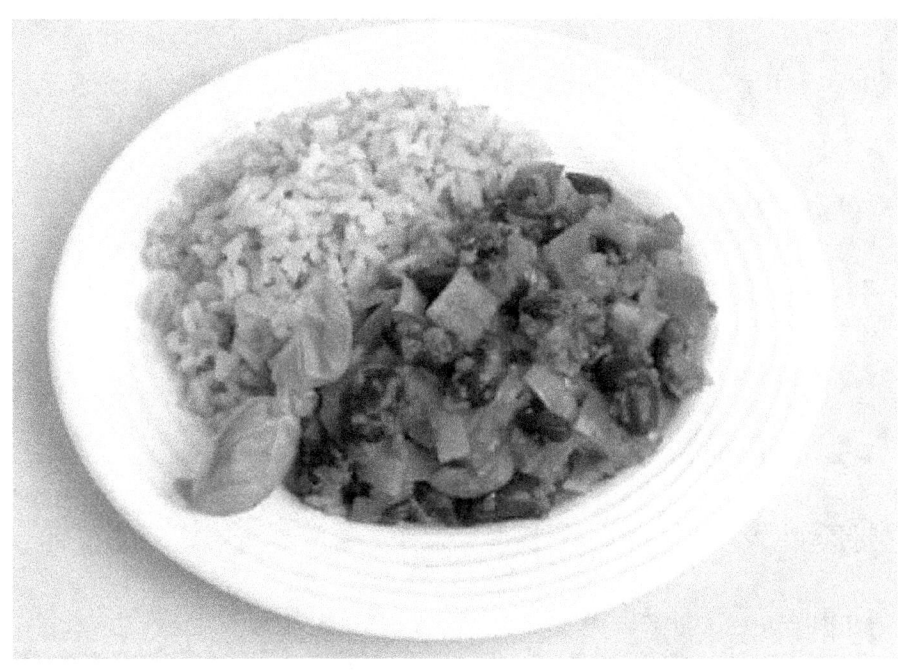

South Asian Masala Paratha

(Ready in about 20 minutes | Servings 5)

Per serving : Calories: 441; Fat: 30.4g; Carbs: 38.1g; Protein: 5.2g

Ingredients

2 cups all-purpose flour

1 teaspoon Kala namak salt

1/2 teaspoon garam masala

1/2 cup warm water

1 tablespoon canola oil

10 tablespoons coconut oil, softened

Directions

In a mixing bowl, thoroughly combine the flour, salt and garam masala. Make a well in the flour mixture and gradually add in the water and canola oil; mix to combine.

Knead the dough until it forms a sticky ball. Let it rest in your refrigerator overnight.

Divide the dough into 5 equal balls and roll them out on a clean surface. Spread the coconut oil all over the paratha and fold it in half. Spread the coconut oil over it and fold it again.

Roll each paratha into a circle approximately 8 inches in diameter.

Heat a griddle until hot. Cook each paratha for about 3 minutes or until bubbles form on the surface. Turn over and cook on the other side for 3 minutes longer. Serve warm.

Traditional Swedish Raggmunk

(Ready in about 30 minutes | Servings 5)

Per serving : Calories: 356; Fat: 22.1g; Carbs: 36.5g; Protein: 4.3g

Ingredients

1 ½ pounds waxy potatoes, peeled, grated and squeezed

3 tablespoons shallots, chopped

2 chia eggs

1/2 cup all-purpose flour

1 teaspoon baking powder

Sea salt and ground black, to season

1 teaspoon cayenne pepper

1/2 cup canola oil

6 tablespoons applesauce

Directions

Thoroughly combine the grated potatoes, shallots, chia eggs, flour, baking powder, salt, black pepper and cayenne pepper.

Preheat the oil in a frying pan over a moderate heat.

Spoon 1/4 cup of the potato mixture into the pan and cook the potato cakes for about 5 minutes per side. Repeat with the remaining batter.

Serve with applesauce and enjoy!

Buffalo Gravy with Beer

(Ready in about 30 minutes | Servings 5)

Per serving : Calories: 222; Fat: 16.8g; Carbs: 11.2g; Protein: 7.3g

Ingredients

3 tablespoons olive oil

1 small red onion, chopped

1 teaspoon garlic, minced

1/3 cup whole wheat flour

3 cups vegetable broth

1/2 teaspoon dried rosemary

1/2 teaspoon dried oregano

1/2 teaspoon dried parsley flakes

1/2 teaspoon dried sage

1 teaspoon hot paprika

Sea salt and freshly cracked black peppercorns, to taste

1 cup beer

Directions

Heat the olive oil in a large saucepan over medium-high heat. Once hot, sauté the onion and garlic until tender and fragrant.

Add in the flour and continue to cook for 1 minute more.

Pour in the vegetable broth and bring to a boil over medium-high heat; stir in the spices and turn the heat to a simmer.

Pour in the beer and let it simmer, partially covered, for about 10 minutes until everything is cooked through.

Serve with mashed potatoes or cauliflower. Bon appétit!

Spicy Cilantro and Mint Chutney

(Ready in about 10 minutes | Servings 9)

Per serving : Calories: 15; Fat: 0g; Carbs: 0.9g; Protein: 0.1g

Ingredients

1 ½ bunches fresh cilantro

6 tablespoons scallions, sliced

3 tablespoons fresh mint leaves

2 jalapeno peppers, seeded

1/2 teaspoon kosher salt

2 tablespoons fresh lime juice

1/3 cup water

Directions

Place all the ingredients in the bowl of your blender or food processor.

Then, combine the ingredients until your desired consistency has been reached.

Bon appétit!

Cinnamon Almond Butter

Ready in about 30 minutes | Servings 16)

Per serving : Calories: 118; Fat: 8.9g; Carbs: 7.5g; Protein: 3.8g

Ingredients

2 cups almonds

1 tablespoon cinnamon, ground

1 teaspoon pure vanilla extract

3 tablespoons agave syrup

A pinch of sea salt

A pinch of grated nutmeg

Directions

Roast the almonds in the preheated oven at 350 degrees F for approximately 9 minutes until your nuts are fragrant and lightly browned.

In your food processor or a high-speed blender, pulse the almonds until ground. Then, process the mixture for 10 minutes more, scraping down the sides and bottom of the bowl.

Add in the cinnamon, vanilla, agave syrup, salt and nutmeg.

Run your machine for another 10 minutes or until your butter is completely creamy and smooth. Enjoy!

Rainbow Vegetable Pancakes

(Ready in about 20 minutes | Servings 4)

Per serving : Calories: 222; Fat: 4.9g; Carbs: 38.1g; Protein: 7.5g

Ingredients

1 cup all-purpose flour

1 teaspoon baking powder

Sea salt and ground black pepper, to taste

1 teaspoon paprika

1 cup zucchini, grated

1 cup button mushrooms, chopped

2 medium carrots, trimmed and grated

1 red onion, finely chopped

1 garlic clove, minced

1 cup spinach, torn into pieces

1/4 cup water

1 teaspoon hot sauce

2 chia eggs

Directions

Thoroughly combine the flour, baking powder, salt, black pepper and paprika. In a separate bowl, combine the vegetables and water.

Add in the hot sauce and chia eggs and mix to combine well. Add the vegetable mixture to the dry flour mixture; stir to combine well.

Then, heat the oil in a frying pan over a moderate flame. Cook the pancakes for 2 to 3 minutes per side until crispy and golden brown.

Bon appétit!

Garden Tomato Relish

(Ready in about 10 minutes + chilling time | Servings 10)

Per serving : Calories: 208; Fat: 21.8g; Carbs: 3.5g; Protein: 0.7g

Ingredients

1 pound tomatoes, chopped

1 red onion, chopped

1 garlic clove, minced

1 cup extra-virgin olive oil

2 tablespoons capers

1 teaspoon chili powder

1 tablespoon curry powder

2 tablespoons cilantro, chopped

2 tablespoons malt vinegar

Directions

Thoroughly combine the tomatoes, onion, garlic and olive oil. Grill for about 8 minutes.

Add in the remaining ingredients and stir to combine well.

Transfer the relish to a bowl and place, uncovered, in your refrigerator for about 2 hours. Bon appétit!

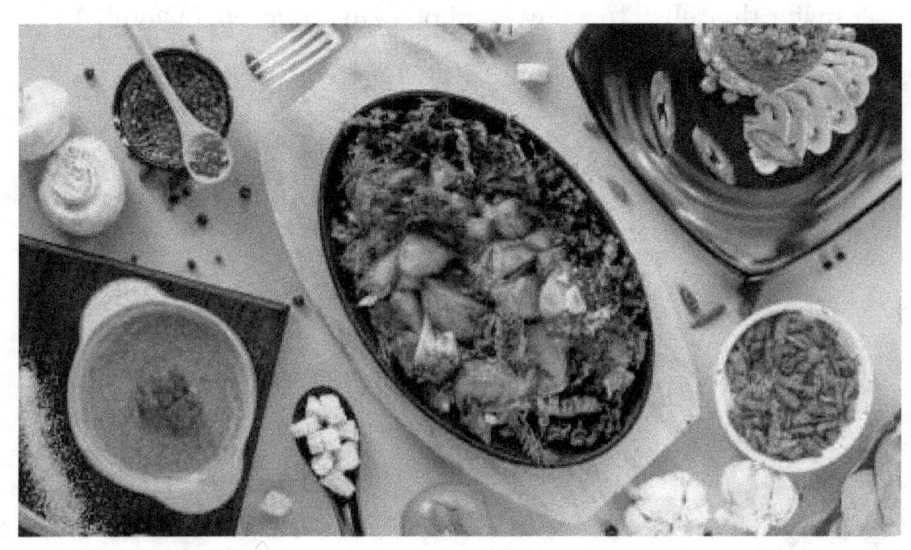

Crunchy Peanut Butter

(Ready in about 10 minutes | Servings 20)

Per serving : Calories: 114; Fat: 9g; Carbs: 5.6g; Protein: 4.8g

Ingredients

2 ½ cups peanuts

1/2 teaspoon coarse sea salt

1/2 teaspoon cinnamon powder

10 dates, pitted

Directions

Roast the peanuts in the preheated oven at 350 degrees F for approximately 7 minutes until the peanuts are fragrant and lightly browned.

In your food processor or a high-speed blender, pulse the peanuts until ground. Reserve for about 1/2 cup of the mixture.

Then, process the mixture for 2 minutes more, scraping down the sides and bottom of the bowl.

Add in the salt, cinnamon and dates.

Run your machine for another 2 minutes or until your butter is smooth. Add in the reserved peanuts and stir with a spoon. Enjoy!

Easy Orange Butter

(Ready in about 10 minutes | Servings 7)

Per serving : Calories: 140; Fat: 13.6g; Carbs: 6.3g; Protein: 0g

Ingredients

2 tablespoons granulated sugar

2 tablespoons cornstarch

1 teaspoon orange zest

1 teaspoon fresh ginger, peeled and minced

2 tablespoons orange juice

1/2 cup water

A pinch of grated nutmeg

A pinch of grated kosher salt

7 tablespoons coconut oil, softened

Directions

In a saucepan, combine the sugar, cornstarch, orange zest and ginger over a moderate heat.

Stir in the orange juice, water, nutmeg and salt; continue to cook until the mixture has thickened. Heat off.

Stir in the coconut oil. Bon appétit!

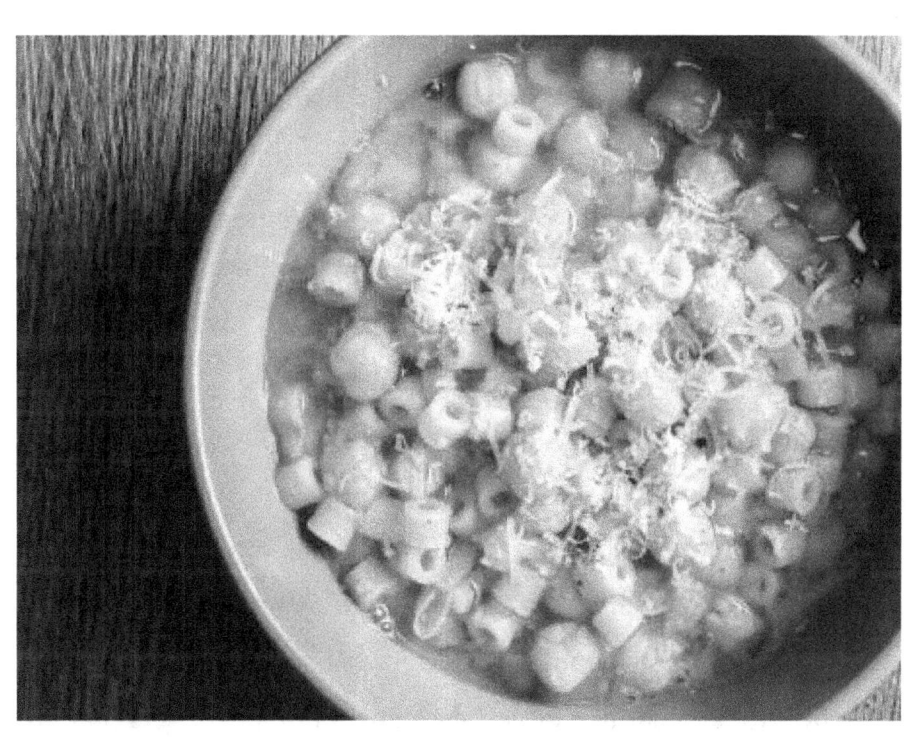

Introduciton

It is only until recently that more and more people are starting to embrace the plant-based diet lifestyle. As to what exactly has drawn tens of millions of people into this lifestyle is debatable. However, there is growing evidence demonstrating that following a primarily plant-based diet lifestyle leads to better weight control and general health, free of many chronic diseases. What are the Health Benefits of a Plant-Based Diet? As it turns out, eating plant-based is one of the healthiest diets in the world. Healthy vegan diets include plenty of fresh products, whole grains, legumes, and healthy fats such as seeds and nuts. They are abundant with antioxidants, minerals, vitamins, and dietary fiber. Current scientific researches pointed out that higher consumption of plant-based foods is associated with a lower risk of mortality from conditions such as cardiovascular disease, type 2 diabetes, hypertension, and obesity. Vegan eating plans often rely heavily on healthy staples, avoiding animal products that are loaded with antibiotics, additives, and hormones. Plus, consuming a higher proportion of essential amino acids with animal protein can be damaging to human health. Since animal products contain much 8 more fat than plant-based foods, it's not a shocker that studies have shown that meat-eaters have nine times the obesity rate of vegans. This leads us to the next point, one of the greatest benefits of the vegan diet – weight loss. While many people choose to live a vegan life for ethical reasons, the diet itself can help you achieve your weight loss goals. If you're struggling to shift pounds, you may want to consider trying a plant-based diet. How exactly? As a vegan, you will reduce the number of high-calorie foods such as full-fat dairy products, fatty fish, pork and other cholesterol containing foods such as eggs. Try replacing such foods with high fiber and protein-rich alternatives that will keep you fuller longer. The key is focusing on nutrient-dense, clean and natural foods and avoid empty calories such as sugar, saturated fats, and highly processed foods. Here are a few tricks that help me maintain my weight on the vegan diet for years. I eat vegetables as a main course; I consume good fats in moderation – a good fat such as olive oil does not make you fat; I exercise regularly and cook at home. Enjoy!

LEGUMES

Traditional Indian Rajma Dal

(Ready in about 20 minutes | Servings 4)

Per serving : Calories: 269; Fat: 15.2g; Carbs: 22.9g; Protein: 7.2g

Ingredients

3 tablespoons sesame oil

1 teaspoon ginger, minced

1 teaspoon cumin seeds

1 teaspoon coriander seeds

1 large onion, chopped

1 celery stalk, chopped

1 teaspoon garlic, minced

1 cup tomato sauce

1 teaspoon garam masala

1/2 teaspoon curry powder

1 small cinnamon stick

1 green chili, seeded and minced

2 cups canned red kidney beans, drained

2 cups vegetable broth

Kosher salt and ground black pepper, to taste

Directions

In a saucepan, heat the sesame oil over medium-high heat; now, sauté the ginger, cumin seeds and coriander seeds until fragrant or about 30 seconds or so.

Add in the onion and celery and continue to sauté for 3 minutes more until they've softened.

Add in the garlic and continue to sauté for 1 minute longer.

Stir the remaining ingredients into the saucepan and turn the heat to a simmer. Continue to cook for 10 to 12 minutes or until thoroughly cooked. Serve warm and enjoy!

Red Kidney Bean Salad

(Ready in about 1 hour + chilling time | Servings 6)

Per serving : Calories: 443; Fat: 19.2g; Carbs: 52.2g; Protein: 18.1g

Ingredients

3/4 pound red kidney beans, soaked overnight

2 bell peppers, chopped

1 carrot, trimmed and grated

3 ounces frozen or canned corn kernels, drained

3 heaping tablespoons scallions, chopped

2 cloves garlic, minced

1 red chile pepper, sliced

1/2 cup extra-virgin olive oil

2 tablespoons apple cider vinegar

2 tablespoons fresh lemon juice

Sea salt and ground black pepper, to taste

2 tablespoons fresh cilantro, chopped

2 tablespoons fresh parsley, chopped

2 tablespoons fresh basil, chopped

Directions

Cover the soaked beans with a fresh change of cold water and bring to a boil. Let it boil for about 10 minutes. Turn the heat to a simmer and continue to cook for 50 to 55 minutes or until tender.

Allow your beans to cool completely, then, transfer them to a salad bowl.

Add in the remaining ingredients and toss to combine well. Bon appétit!

Anasazi Bean and Vegetable Stew

(Ready in about 1 hour | Servings 3)

Per serving : Calories: 444; Fat: 15.8g; Carbs: 58.2g; Protein: 20.2g

Ingredients

1 cup Anasazi beans, soaked overnight and drained

3 cups roasted vegetable broth

1 bay laurel

1 thyme sprig, chopped

1 rosemary sprig, chopped

3 tablespoons olive oil

1 large onion, chopped

2 celery stalks, chopped

2 carrots, chopped

2 bell peppers, seeded and chopped

1 green chili pepper, seeded and chopped

2 garlic cloves, minced

Sea salt and ground black pepper, to taste

1 teaspoon cayenne pepper

1 teaspoon paprika

Directions

In a saucepan, bring the Anasazi beans and broth to a boil. Once boiling, turn the heat to a simmer. Add in the bay laurel, thyme and rosemary; let it cook for about 50 minutes or until tender.

Meanwhile, in a heavy-bottomed pot, heat the olive oil over medium-high heat. Now, sauté the onion, celery, carrots and peppers for about 4 minutes until tender.

Add in the garlic and continue to sauté for 30 seconds more or until aromatic.

Add the sautéed mixture to the cooked beans. Season with salt, black pepper, cayenne pepper and paprika.

Continue to simmer, stirring periodically, for 10 minutes more or until everything is cooked through. Bon appétit!

Easy and Hearty Shakshuka

(Ready in about 50 minutes | Servings 4)

Per serving : Calories: 324; Fat: 11.2g; Carbs: 42.2g; Protein: 15.8g

Ingredients

2 tablespoons olive oil

1 onion, chopped

2 bell peppers, chopped

1 poblano pepper, chopped

2 cloves garlic, minced

2 tomatoes, pureed

Sea salt and black pepper, to taste

1 teaspoon dried basil

1 teaspoon red pepper flakes

1 teaspoon paprika

2 bay leaves

1 cup chickpeas, soaked overnight, rinsed and drained

3 cups vegetable broth

2 tablespoons fresh cilantro, roughly chopped

Directions

Heat the olive oil in a saucepan over medium heat. Once hot, cook the onion, peppers and garlic for about 4 minutes, until tender and aromatic.

Add in the pureed tomato tomatoes, sea salt, black pepper, basil, red pepper, paprika and bay leaves.

Turn the heat to a simmer and add in the chickpeas and vegetable broth. Cook for 45 minutes or until tender.

Taste and adjust seasonings. Spoon your shakshuka into individual bowls and serve garnished with the fresh cilantro. Bon appétit!

Old-Fashioned Chili

(Ready in about 1 hour 30 minutes | Servings 4)

Per serving : Calories: 514; Fat: 16.4g; Carbs: 72g; Protein: 25.8g

Ingredients

3/4 pound red kidney beans, soaked overnight

2 tablespoons olive oil

1 onion, chopped

2 bell peppers, chopped

1 red chili pepper, chopped

2 ribs celery, chopped

2 cloves garlic, minced

2 bay leaves

1 teaspoon ground cumin

1 teaspoon thyme, chopped

1 teaspoon black peppercorns

20 ounces tomatoes, crushed

2 cups vegetable broth

1 teaspoon smoked paprika

Sea salt, to taste

2 tablespoons fresh cilantro, chopped

1 avocado, pitted, peeled and sliced

Directions

Cover the soaked beans with a fresh change of cold water and bring to a boil. Let it boil for about 10 minutes. Turn the heat to a simmer and continue to cook for 50 to 55 minutes or until tender.

In a heavy-bottomed pot, heat the olive oil over medium heat. Once hot, sauté the onion, bell pepper and celery.

Sauté the garlic, bay leaves, ground cumin, thyme and black peppercorns for about 1 minute or so.

Add in the diced tomatoes, vegetable broth, paprika, salt and cooked beans. Let it simmer, stirring periodically, for 25 to 30 minutes or until cooked through.

Serve garnished with fresh cilantro and avocado. Bon appétit!

Easy Red Lentil Salad

(Ready in about 20 minutes + chilling time | Servings 3)

Per serving : Calories: 295; Fat: 18.8g; Carbs: 25.2g; Protein: 8.5g

Ingredients

1/2 cup red lentils, soaked overnight and drained

1 ½ cups water

1 sprig rosemary

1 bay leaf

1 cup grape tomatoes, halved

1 cucumber, thinly sliced

1 bell pepper, thinly sliced

1 clove garlic, minced

1 onion, thinly sliced

2 tablespoons fresh lime juice

4 tablespoons olive oil

Sea salt and ground black pepper, to taste

Directions

Add the red lentils, water, rosemary and bay leaf to a saucepan and bring to a boil over high heat. Then, turn the heat to a simmer and continue to cook for 20 minutes or until tender.

Place the lentils in a salad bowl and let them cool completely.

Add in the remaining ingredients and toss to combine well. Serve at room temperature or well-chilled.

Bon appétit!

Mediterranean-Style Chickpea Salad

(Ready in about 40 minutes + chilling time | Servings 4)

Per serving : Calories: 468; Fat: 12.5g; Carbs: 73g; Protein: 21.8g

Ingredients

2 cups chickpeas, soaked overnight and drained

1 Persian cucumber, sliced

1 cup cherry tomatoes, halved

1 red bell peppers, seeded and sliced

1 green bell pepper, seeded and sliced

1 teaspoon deli mustard

1 teaspoon coriander seeds

1 teaspoon jalapeno pepper, minced

1 tablespoon fresh lemon juice

1 tablespoon balsamic vinegar

1/4 cup extra-virgin olive oil

Sea salt and ground black pepper, to taste

2 tablespoons fresh cilantro, chopped

2 tablespoons Kalamata olives, pitted and sliced

Directions

Place the chickpeas in a stockpot; cover the chickpeas with water by 2 inches. Bring it to a boil.

Immediately turn the heat to a simmer and continue to cook for about 40 minutes or until tender.

Transfer your chickpeas to a salad bowl. Add in the remaining ingredients and toss to combine well. Bon appétit!

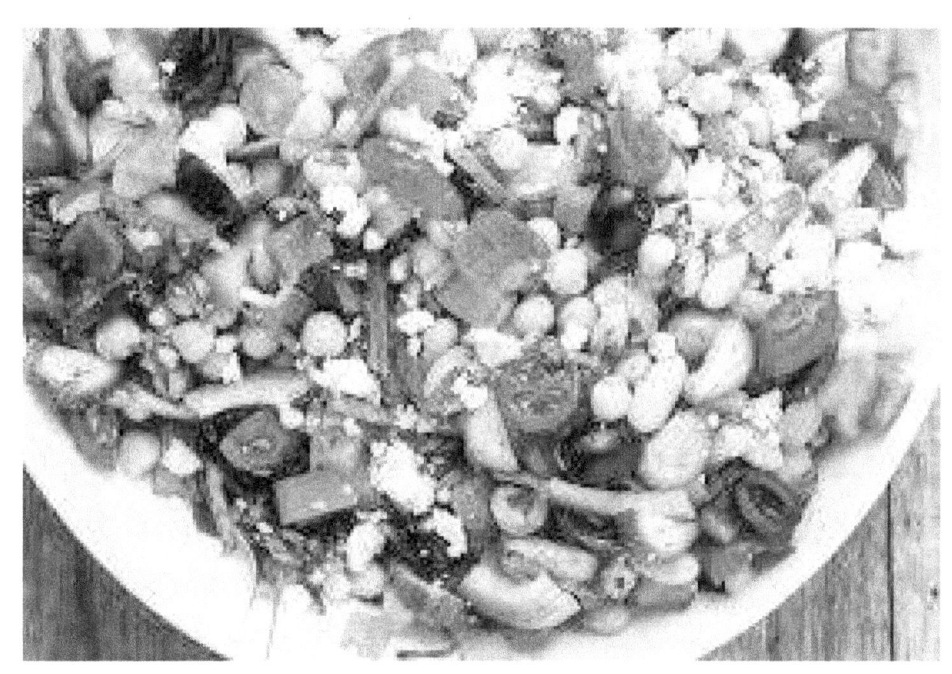

Traditional Tuscan Bean Stew (Ribollita)

(Ready in about 25 minutes | Servings 5)

Per serving : Calories: 388; Fat: 10.3g; Carbs: 57.3g; Protein: 19.5g

Ingredients

3 tablespoons olive oil

1 medium leek, chopped

1 celery with leaves, chopped

1 zucchini, diced

1 Italian pepper, sliced

3 garlic cloves, crushed

2 bay leaves

Kosher salt and ground black pepper, to taste

1 teaspoon cayenne pepper

1 (28-ounce) can tomatoes, crushed

2 cups vegetable broth

2 (15-ounce) cans Great Northern beans, drained

2 cups Lacinato kale, torn into pieces

1 cup crostini

Directions

In a heavy-bottomed pot, heat the olive oil over medium heat. Once hot, sauté the leek, celery, zucchini and pepper for about 4 minutes.

Sauté the garlic and bay leaves for about 1 minute or so.

Add in the spices, tomatoes, broth and canned beans. Let it simmer, stirring occasionally, for about 15 minutes or until cooked through.

Add in the Lacinato kale and continue simmering, stirring occasionally, for 4 minutes.

Serve garnished with crostini. Bon appétit!

Beluga Lentil and Vegetable Mélange

(Ready in about 25 minutes | Servings 5)

Per serving : Calories: 382; Fat: 9.3g; Carbs: 59g; Protein: 17.2g

Ingredients

3 tablespoons olive oil

1 onion, minced

2 bell peppers, seeded and chopped

1 carrot, trimmed and chopped

1 parsnip, trimmed and chopped

1 teaspoon ginger, minced

2 cloves garlic, minced

Sea salt and ground black pepper, to taste

1 large-sized zucchini, diced

1 cup tomato sauce

1 cup vegetable broth

1 ½ cups beluga lentils, soaked overnight and drained

2 cups Swiss chard

Directions

In a Dutch oven, heat the olive oil until sizzling. Now, sauté the onion, bell pepper, carrot and parsnip, until they've softened.

Add in the ginger and garlic and continue sautéing an additional 30 seconds.

Now, add in the salt, black pepper, zucchini, tomato sauce, vegetable broth and lentils; let it simmer for about 20 minutes until everything is thoroughly cooked.

Add in the Swiss chard; cover and let it simmer for 5 minutes more. Bon appétit!

Mexican Chickpea Taco Bowls

(Ready in about 15 minutes | Servings 4)

Per serving : Calories: 409; Fat: 13.5g; Carbs: 61.3g; Protein: 13.8g

Ingredients

2 tablespoons sesame oil

1 red onion, chopped

1 habanero pepper, minced

2 garlic cloves, crushed

2 bell peppers, seeded and diced

Sea salt and ground black pepper

1/2 teaspoon Mexican oregano

1 teaspoon ground cumin

2 ripe tomatoes, pureed

1 teaspoon brown sugar

16 ounces canned chickpeas, drained

4 (8-inch) flour tortillas

2 tablespoons fresh coriander, roughly chopped

Directions

In a large skillet, heat the sesame oil over a moderately high heat. Then, sauté the onions for 2 to 3 minutes or until tender.

Add in the peppers and garlic and continue to sauté for 1 minute or until fragrant.

Add in the spices, tomatoes and brown sugar and bring to a boil. Immediately turn the heat to a simmer, add in the canned chickpeas and let it cook for 8 minutes longer or until heated through.

Toast your tortillas and arrange them with the prepared chickpea mixture.

Top with fresh coriander and serve immediately. Bon appétit!

Indian Dal Makhani

(Ready in about 20 minutes | Servings 6)

Per serving : Calories: 329; Fat: 8.5g; Carbs: 44.1g; Protein: 16.8g

Ingredients

3 tablespoons sesame oil

1 large onion, chopped

1 bell pepper, seeded and chopped

2 garlic cloves, minced

1 tablespoon ginger, grated

2 green chilies, seeded and chopped

1 teaspoon cumin seeds

1 bay laurel

1 teaspoon turmeric powder

1/4 teaspoon red peppers

1/4 teaspoon ground allspice

1/2 teaspoon garam masala

1 cup tomato sauce

4 cups vegetable broth

1 ½ cups black lentils, soaked overnight and drained

4-5 curry leaves, for garnis h

Directions

In a saucepan, heat the sesame oil over medium-high heat; now, sauté the onion and bell pepper for 3 minutes more until they've softened.

Add in the garlic, ginger, green chilies, cumin seeds and bay laurel; continue to sauté, stirring frequently, for 1 minute or until fragrant.

Stir in the remaining ingredients, except for the curry leaves. Now, turn the heat to a simmer. Continue to cook for 15 minutes more or until thoroughly cooked.

Garnish with curry leaves and serve hot!

Mexican-Style Bean Bowl

(Ready in about 1 hour + chilling time | Servings 6)

Per serving : Calories: 465; Fat: 17.9g; Carbs: 60.4g; Protein: 20.2g

Ingredients

1 pound red beans, soaked overnight and drained

1 cup canned corn kernels, drained

2 roasted bell peppers, sliced

1 chili pepper, finely chopped

1 cup cherry tomatoes, halved

1 red onion, chopped

1/4 cup fresh cilantro, chopped

1/4 cup fresh parsley, chopped

1 teaspoon Mexican oregano

1/4 cup red wine vinegar

2 tablespoons fresh lemon juice

1/3 cup extra-virgin olive oil

Sea salt and ground black, to taste

1 avocado, peeled, pitted and sliced

Directions

Cover the soaked beans with a fresh change of cold water and bring to a boil. Let it boil for about 10 minutes. Turn the heat to a simmer and continue to cook for 50 to 55 minutes or until tender.

Allow your beans to cool completely, then, transfer them to a salad bowl.

Add in the remaining ingredients and toss to combine well. Serve at room temperature.

Bon appétit!

Classic Italian Minestrone

(Ready in about 30 minutes | Servings 5)

Per serving : Calories: 305; Fat: 8.6g; Carbs: 45.1g; Protein: 14.2g

Ingredients

2 tablespoons olive oil

1 large onion, diced

2 carrots, sliced

4 cloves garlic, minced

1 cup elbow pasta

5 cups vegetable broth

1 (15-ounce) can white beans, drained

1 large zucchini, diced

1 (28-ounce) can tomatoes, crushed

1 tablespoon fresh oregano leaves, chopped

1 tablespoon fresh basil leaves, chopped

1 tablespoon fresh Italian parsley, chopped

Directions

In a Dutch oven, heat the olive oil until sizzling. Now, sauté the onion and carrots until they've softened.

Add in the garlic, uncooked pasta and broth; let it simmer for about 15 minutes.

Stir in the beans, zucchini, tomatoes and herbs. Continue to cook, covered, for about 10 minutes until everything is thoroughly cooked.

Garnish with some extra herbs, if desired. Bon appétit!

Green Lentil Stew with Collard Greens

(Ready in about 30 minutes | Servings 5)

Per serving : Calories: 415; Fat: 6.6g; Carbs: 71g; Protein: 18.4g

Ingredients

2 tablespoons olive oil

1 onion, chopped

2 sweet potatoes, peeled and diced

1 bell pepper, chopped

2 carrots, chopped

1 parsnip, chopped

1 celery, chopped

2 cloves garlic

1 ½ cups green lentils

1 tablespoon Italian herb mix

1 cup tomato sauce

5 cups vegetable broth

1 cup frozen corn

1 cup collard greens, torn into pieces

Directions

In a Dutch oven, heat the olive oil until sizzling. Now, sauté the onion, sweet potatoes, bell pepper, carrots, parsnip and celery until they've softened.

Add in the garlic and continue sautéing an additional 30 seconds.

Now, add in the green lentils, Italian herb mix, tomato sauce and vegetable broth; let it simmer for about 20 minutes until everything is thoroughly cooked.

Add in the frozen corn and collard greens; cover and let it simmer for 5 minutes more. Bon appétit!

Chickpea Garden Vegetable Medley

(Ready in about 30 minutes | Servings 4)

Per serving : Calories: 369; Fat: 18.1g; Carbs: 43.5g; Protein: 13.2g

Ingredients

2 tablespoons olive oil

1 onion, finely chopped

1 bell pepper, chopped

1 fennel bulb, chopped

3 cloves garlic, minced

2 ripe tomatoes, pureed

2 tablespoons fresh parsley, roughly chopped

2 tablespoons fresh basil, roughly chopped

2 tablespoons fresh coriander, roughly chopped

2 cups vegetable broth

14 ounces canned chickpeas, drained

Kosher salt and ground black pepper, to taste

1/2 teaspoon cayenne pepper

1 teaspoon paprika

1 avocado, peeled and sliced

Directions

In a heavy-bottomed pot, heat the olive oil over medium heat. Once hot, sauté the onion, bell pepper and fennel bulb for about 4 minutes.

Sauté the garlic for about 1 minute or until aromatic.

Add in the tomatoes, fresh herbs, broth, chickpeas, salt, black pepper, cayenne pepper and paprika. Let it simmer, stirring occasionally, for about 20 minutes or until cooked through.

Taste and adjust the seasonings. Serve garnished with the slices of the fresh avocado. Bon appétit!

Hot Bean Dipping Sauce

(Ready in about 30 minutes | Servings 10)

Per serving : Calories: 175; Fat: 4.7g; Carbs: 24.9g; Protein: 8.8g

Ingredients

2 (15-ounce) cans Great Northern beans, drained

2 tablespoons olive oil

2 tablespoons Sriracha sauce

2 tablespoons nutritional yeast

4 ounces vegan cream cheese

1/2 teaspoon paprika

1/2 teaspoon cayenne pepper

1/2 teaspoon ground cumin

Sea salt and ground black pepper, to taste

4 ounces tortilla chips

Directions

Start by preheating your oven to 360 degrees F.

Pulse all the ingredients, except for the tortilla chips, in your food processor until your desired consistency is reached.

Bake your dip in the preheated oven for about 25 minutes or until hot.

Serve with tortilla chips and enjoy!

Chinese-Style Soybean Salad

(Ready in about 10 minutes | Servings 4)

Per serving : Calories: 265; Fat: 13.7g; Carbs: 21g; Protein: 18g

Ingredients

1 (15-ounce) can soybeans, drained

1 cup arugula

1 cup baby spinach

1 cup green cabbage, shredded

1 onion, thinly sliced

1/2 teaspoon garlic, minced

1 teaspoon ginger, minced

1/2 teaspoon deli mustard

2 tablespoons soy sauce

1 tablespoon rice vinegar

1 tablespoon lime juice

2 tablespoons tahini

1 teaspoon agave syrup

Directions

In a salad bowl, place the soybeans, arugula, spinach, cabbage and onion; toss to combine.

In a small mixing dish, whisk the remaining ingredients for the dressing.

Dress your salad and serve immediately. Bon appétit!

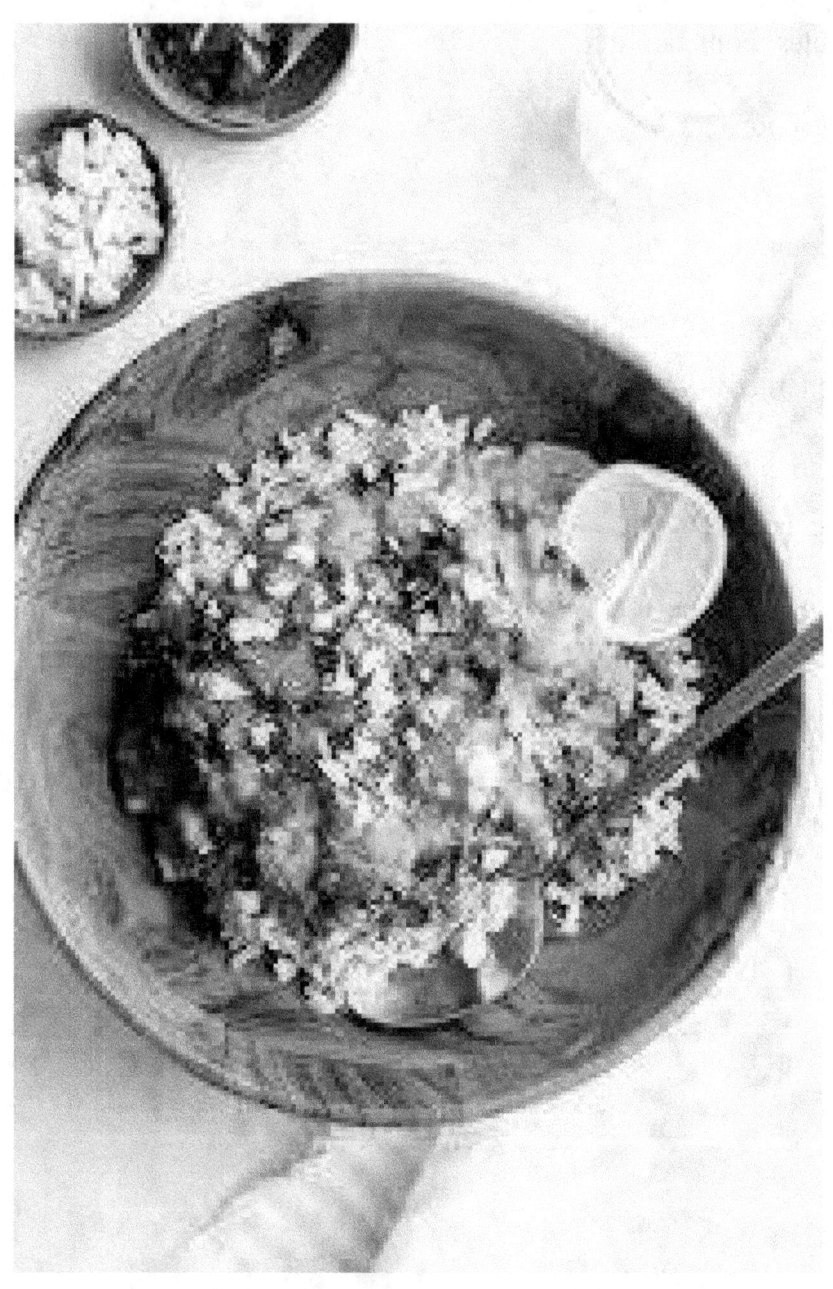

Old-Fashioned Lentil and Vegetable Stew

(Ready in about 25 minutes | Servings 5)

Per serving : Calories: 475; Fat: 17.3g; Carbs: 61.4g; Protein: 23.7g

Ingredients

3 tablespoons olive oil

1 large onion, chopped

1 carrot, chopped

1 bell pepper, diced

1 habanero pepper, chopped

3 cloves garlic, minced

Kosher salt and black pepper, to taste

1 teaspoon ground cumin

1 teaspoon smoked paprika

1 (28-ounce) can tomatoes, crushed

2 tablespoons tomato ketchup

4 cups vegetable broth

3/4 pound dry red lentils, soaked overnight and drained

1 avocado, sliced

Directions

In a heavy-bottomed pot, heat the olive oil over medium heat. Once hot, sauté the onion, carrot and peppers for about 4 minutes.

Sauté the garlic for about 1 minute or so.

Add in the spices, tomatoes, ketchup, broth and canned lentils. Let it simmer, stirring occasionally, for about 20 minutes or until cooked through.

Serve garnished with the slices of avocado. Bon appétit!

Indian Chana Masala

(Ready in about 15 minutes | Servings 4)

Per serving : Calories: 305; Fat: 17.1g; Carbs: 30.1g; Protein: 9.4g

Ingredients

1 cup tomatoes, pureed

1 Kashmiri chile pepper, chopped

1 large shallot, chopped

1 teaspoon fresh ginger, peeled and grated

4 tablespoons olive oil

2 cloves garlic, minced

1 teaspoon coriander seeds

1 teaspoon garam masala

1/2 teaspoon turmeric powder

Sea salt and ground black pepper, to taste

1/2 cup vegetable broth

16 ounces canned chickpeas

1 tablespoon fresh lime juice

Directions

In your blender or food processor, blend the tomatoes, Kashmiri chile pepper, shallot and ginger into a paste.

In a saucepan, heat the olive oil over medium heat. Once hot, cook the prepared paste and garlic for about 2 minutes.

Add in the remaining spices, broth and chickpeas. Turn the heat to a simmer. Continue to simmer for 8 minutes more or until cooked through.

Remove from the heat. Drizzle fresh lime juice over the top of each serving. Bon appétit!

Red Kidney Bean Pâté

(Ready in about 10 minutes | Servings 8)

Per serving : Calories: 135; Fat: 12.1g; Carbs: 4.4g; Protein: 1.6g

Ingredients

2 tablespoons olive oil

1 onion, chopped

1 bell pepper, chopped

2 cloves garlic, minced

2 cups red kidney beans, boiled and drained

1/4 cup olive oil

1 teaspoon stone-ground mustard

2 tablespoons fresh parsley, chopped

2 tablespoons fresh basil, chopped

Sea salt and ground black pepper, to taste

Directions

In a saucepan, heat the olive oil over medium-high heat. Now, cook the onion, pepper and garlic until just tender or about 3 minutes.

Add the sautéed mixture to your blender; add in the remaining ingredients. Puree the ingredients in your blender or food processor until smooth and creamy.

Bon appétit!

Brown Lentil Bowl

(Ready in about 20 minutes + chilling time | Servings 4)

Per serving : Calories: 452; Fat: 16.6g; Carbs: 61.7g; Protein: 16.4g

Ingredients

1 cup brown lentils, soaked overnight and drained

3 cups water

2 cups brown rice, cooked

1 zucchini, diced

1 red onion, chopped

1 teaspoon garlic, minced

1 cucumber, sliced

1 bell pepper, sliced

4 tablespoons olive oil

1 tablespoon rice vinegar

2 tablespoons lemon juice

2 tablespoons soy sauce

1/2 teaspoon dried oregano

1/2 teaspoon ground cumin

Sea salt and ground black pepper, to taste

2 cups arugula

2 cups Romaine lettuce, torn into pieces

Directions

Add the brown lentils and water to a saucepan and bring to a boil over high heat. Then, turn the heat to a simmer and continue to cook for 20 minutes or until tender.

Place the lentils in a salad bowl and let them cool completely.

Add in the remaining ingredients and toss to combine well. Serve at room temperature or well-chilled. Bon appétit!

Hot and Spicy Anasazi Bean Soup

(Ready in about 1 hour 10 minutes | Servings 5)

Per serving : Calories: 352; Fat: 8.5g; Carbs: 50.1g; Protein: 19.7g

Ingredients

2 cups Anasazi beans, soaked overnight, drained and rinsed

8 cups water

2 bay leaves

3 tablespoons olive oil

2 medium onions, chopped

2 bell peppers, chopped

1 habanero pepper, chopped

3 cloves garlic, pressed or minced

Sea salt and ground black pepper, to taste

Directions

In a soup pot, bring the Anasazi beans and water to a boil. Once boiling, turn the heat to a simmer. Add in the bay leaves and let it cook for about 1 hour or until tender.

Meanwhile, in a heavy-bottomed pot, heat the olive oil over medium-high heat. Now, sauté the onion, peppers and garlic for about 4 minutes until tender.

Add the sautéed mixture to the cooked beans. Season with salt and black pepper.

Continue to simmer, stirring periodically, for 10 minutes more or until everything is cooked through. Bon appétit!

Black-Eyed Pea Salad (Ñebbe)

(Ready in about 1 hour | Servings 5)

Per serving : Calories: 471; Fat: 17.5g; Carbs: 61.5g; Protein: 20.6g

Ingredients

2 cups dried black-eyed peas, soaked overnight and drained

2 tablespoons basil leaves, chopped

2 tablespoons parsley leaves, chopped

1 shallot, chopped

1 cucumber, sliced

2 bell peppers, seeded and diced

1 Scotch bonnet chili pepper, seeded and finely chopped

1 cup cherry tomatoes, quartered

Sea salt and ground black pepper, to taste

2 tablespoons fresh lime juice

1 tablespoon apple cider vinegar

1/4 cup extra-virgin olive oil

1 avocado, peeled, pitted and sliced

Directions

Cover the black-eyed peas with water by 2 inches and bring to a gentle boil. Let it boil for about 15 minutes.

Then, turn the heat to a simmer for about 45 minutes. Let it cool completely.

Place the black-eyed peas in a salad bowl. Add in the basil, parsley, shallot, cucumber, bell peppers, cherry tomatoes, salt and black pepper.

In a mixing bowl, whisk the lime juice, vinegar and olive oil.

Dress the salad, garnish with fresh avocado and serve immediately. Bon appétit!

Mom's Famous Chili

(Ready in about 1 hour 30 minutes | Servings 5)

Per serving : Calories: 455; Fat: 10.5g; Carbs: 68.6g; Protein: 24.7g

Ingredients

1 pound red black beans, soaked overnight and drained

3 tablespoons olive oil

1 large red onion, diced

2 bell peppers, diced

1 poblano pepper, minced

1 large carrot, trimmed and diced

2 cloves garlic, minced

2 bay leaves

1 teaspoon mixed peppercorns

Kosher salt and cayenne pepper, to taste

1 tablespoon paprika

2 ripe tomatoes, pureed

2 tablespoons tomato ketchup

3 cups vegetable broth

Directions

Cover the soaked beans with a fresh change of cold water and bring to a boil. Let it boil for about 10 minutes. Turn the heat to a simmer and continue to cook for 50 to 55 minutes or until tender.

In a heavy-bottomed pot, heat the olive oil over medium heat. Once hot, sauté the onion, peppers and carrot.

Sauté the garlic for about 30 seconds or until aromatic.

Add in the remaining ingredients along with the cooked beans. Let it simmer, stirring periodically, for 25 to 30 minutes or until cooked through.

Discard the bay leaves, ladle into individual bowls and serve hot!

Creamed Chickpea Salad with Pine Nuts

(Ready in about 10 minutes | Servings 4)

Per serving : Calories: 386; Fat: 22.5g; Carbs: 37.2g; Protein: 12.9g

Ingredients

16 ounces canned chickpeas, drained

1 teaspoon garlic, minced

1 shallot, chopped

1 cup cherry tomatoes, halved

1 bell pepper, seeded and sliced

1/4 cup fresh basil, chopped

1/4 cup fresh parsley, chopped

1/2 cup vegan mayonnaise

1 tablespoon lemon juice

1 teaspoon capers, drained

Sea salt and ground black pepper, to taste

2 ounces pine nuts

Directions

Place the chickpeas, vegetables and herbs in a salad bowl.

Add in the mayonnaise, lemon juice, capers, salt and black pepper. Stir to combine.

Top with pine nuts and serve immediately. Bon appétit!

Black Bean Buda Bowl

(Ready in about 1 hour | Servings 4)

Per serving : Calories: 365; Fat: 14.1g; Carbs: 45.6g; Protein: 15.5g

Ingredients

1/2 pound black beans, soaked overnight and drained

2 cups brown rice, cooked

1 medium-sized onion, thinly sliced

1 cup bell pepper, seeded and sliced

1 jalapeno pepper, seeded and sliced

2 cloves garlic, minced

1 cup arugula

1 cup baby spinach

1 teaspoon lime zest

1 tablespoon Dijon mustard

1/4 cup red wine vinegar

1/4 cup extra-virgin olive oil

2 tablespoons agave syrup

Flaky sea salt and ground black pepper, to taste

1/4 cup fresh Italian parsley, roughly chopped

Directions

Cover the soaked beans with a fresh change of cold water and bring to a boil. Let it boil for about 10 minutes. Turn the heat to a simmer and continue to cook for 50 to 55 minutes or until tender.

To serve, divide the beans and rice between serving bowls; top with the vegetables.

In a small mixing dish, thoroughly combine the lime zest, mustard, vinegar, olive oil, agave syrup, salt and pepper. Drizzle the vinaigrette over the salad.

Garnish with fresh Italian parsley. Bon appétit!

Middle Eastern Chickpea Stew

(Ready in about 20 minutes | Servings 4)

Per serving : Calories: 305; Fat: 11.2g; Carbs: 38.6g; Protein: 12.7g

Ingredients

1 onion, chopped

1 chili pepper, chopped

2 garlic cloves, chopped

1 teaspoon mustard seeds

1 teaspoon coriander seeds

1 bay leaf

1/2 cup tomato puree

2 tablespoons olive oil

1 celery with leaves, chopped

2 medium carrots, trimmed and chopped

2 cups vegetable broth

- 1 teaspoon ground cumin
- 1 small-sized cinnamon stick
- 16 ounces canned chickpeas, drained
- 2 cups Swiss chard, torn into pieces

Directions

In your blender or food processor, blend the onion, chili pepper, garlic, mustard seeds, coriander seeds, bay leaf and tomato puree into a paste.

In a stockpot, heat the olive oil until sizzling. Now, cook the celery and carrots for about 3 minutes or until they've softened. Add in the paste and continue to cook for a further 2 minutes.

Then, add in the vegetable broth, cumin, cinnamon and chickpeas; bring to a gentle boil.

Turn the heat to simmer and let it cook for 6 minutes; fold in Swiss chard and continue to cook for 4 to 5 minutes more or until the leaves wilt. Serve hot and enjoy!

Lentil and Tomato Dip

(Ready in about 10 minutes | Servings 8)

Per serving : Calories: 144; Fat: 4.5g; Carbs: 20.2g; Protein: 8.1g

Ingredients

16 ounces lentils, boiled and drained

4 tablespoons sun-dried tomatoes, chopped

1 cup tomato paste

4 tablespoons tahini

1 teaspoon stone-ground mustard

1 teaspoon ground cumin

1/4 teaspoon ground bay leaf

1 teaspoon red pepper flakes

Sea salt and ground black pepper, to taste

Directions

Blitz all the ingredients in your blender or food processor until your desired consistency is reached.

Place in your refrigerator until ready to serve.

Serve with toasted pita wedges or vegetable sticks. Enjoy!

Creamed Green Pea Salad

(Ready in about 10 minutes + chilling time | Servings 6)

Per serving : Calories: 154; Fat: 6.7g; Carbs: 17.3g; Protein: 6.9g

Ingredients

2 (14.5 ounce) cans green peas, drained

1/2 cup vegan mayonnaise

1 teaspoon Dijon mustard

2 tablespoons scallions, chopped

2 pickles, chopped

1/2 cup marinated mushrooms, chopped and drained

1/2 teaspoon garlic, minced

Sea salt and ground black pepper, to taste

Directions

Place all the ingredients in a salad bowl. Gently stir to combine.

Place the salad in your refrigerator until ready to serve.

Bon appétit!

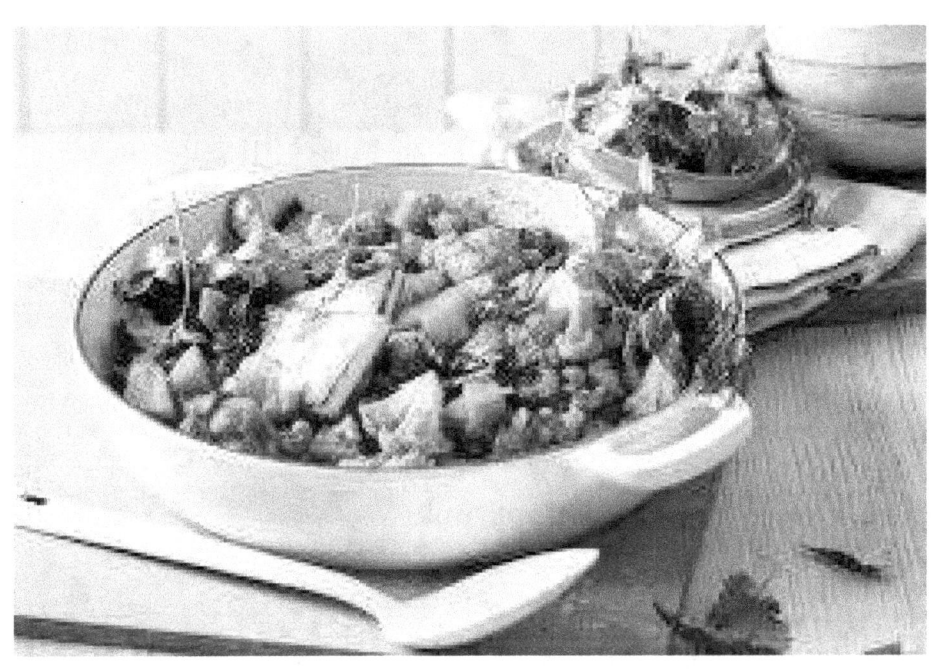

Middle Eastern Za'atar Hummus

(Ready in about 10 minutes | Servings 8)

Per serving : Calories: 140; Fat: 8.5g; Carbs: 12.4g; Protein: 4.6g

Ingredients

10 ounces chickpeas, boiled and drained

1/4 cup tahini

2 tablespoons extra-virgin olive oil

2 tablespoons sun-dried tomatoes, chopped

1 lemon, freshly squeezed

2 garlic cloves, minced

Kosher salt and ground black pepper, to taste

1/2 teaspoon smoked paprika

1 teaspoon Za'atar

Directions

Blitz all the ingredients in your food processor until creamy and uniform.

Place in your refrigerator until ready to serve.

Bon appétit!

Lentil Salad with Pine Nuts

(Ready in about 20 minutes + chilling time | Servings 3)

Per serving : Calories: 332; Fat: 19.7g; Carbs: 28.2g; Protein: 12.2g

Ingredients

1/2 cup brown lentils

1 ½ cups vegetable broth

1 carrot, cut into matchsticks

1 small onion, chopped

1 cucumber, sliced

2 cloves garlic, minced

3 tablespoons extra-virgin olive oil

1 tablespoon red wine vinegar

2 tablespoons lemon juice

2 tablespoons basil, chopped

2 tablespoons parsley, chopped

2 tablespoons chives, chopped

Sea salt and ground black pepper, to taste

2 tablespoons pine nuts, roughly chopped

Directions

Add the brown lentils and vegetable broth to a saucepan and bring to a boil over high heat. Then, turn the heat to a simmer and continue to cook for 20 minutes or until tender.

Place the lentils in a salad bowl.

Add in the vegetables and toss to combine well. In a mixing bowl, whisk the oil, vinegar, lemon juice, basil, parsley, chives, salt and black pepper.

Dress your salad, garnish with pine nuts and serve at room temperature. Bon appétit!

Hot Anasazi Bean Salad

(Ready in about 1 hour | Servings 5)

Per serving : Calories: 482; Fat: 23.1g; Carbs: 54.2g; Protein: 17.2g

Ingredients

2 cups Anasazi beans, soaked overnight, drained and rinsed

6 cups water

1 poblano pepper, chopped

1 onion, chopped

1 cup cherry tomatoes, halved

2 cups mixed greens, ton into pieces

Dressing:

1 teaspoon garlic, chopped

1/2 cup extra-virgin olive oil

1 tablespoon lemon juice

2 tablespoons red wine vinegar

1 tablespoon stone-ground mustard

1 tablespoon soy sauce

1/2 teaspoon dried oregano

1/2 teaspoon dried basil

Sea salt and ground black pepper, to tast e

Directions

In a saucepan, bring the Anasazi beans and water to a boil. Once boiling, turn the heat to a simmer and let it cook for about 1 hour or until tender.

Drain the cooked beans and place them in a salad bowl; add in the other salad ingredients.

Then, in a small mixing bowl, whisk all the dressing ingredients until well blended. Dress your salad and toss to combine. Serve at room temperature and enjoy!

Traditional Mnazaleh Stew

(Ready in about 25 minutes | Servings 4)

Per serving : Calories: 439; Fat: 24g; Carbs: 44.9g; Protein: 13.5g

Ingredients

4 tablespoons olive oil

1 onion, chopped

1 large-sized eggplant, peeled and diced

1 cup carrots, chopped

2 garlic cloves, minced

2 large-sized tomatoes, pureed

1 teaspoon Baharat seasoning

2 cups vegetable broth

14 ounces canned chickpeas, drained

Kosher salt and ground black pepper, to taste

1 medium-sized avocado, pitted, peeled and sliced

Directions

In a heavy-bottomed pot, heat the olive oil over medium heat. Once hot, sauté the onion, eggplant and carrots for about 4 minutes.

Sauté the garlic for about 1 minute or until aromatic.

Add in the tomatoes, Baharat seasoning, broth and canned chickpeas. Let it simmer, stirring occasionally, for about 20 minutes or until cooked through.

Season with salt and pepper. Serve garnished with slices of the fresh avocado. Bon appétit!

Peppery Red Lentil Spread

(Ready in about 25 minutes | Servings 9)

Per serving : Calories: 193; Fat: 8.5g; Carbs: 22.3g; Protein: 8.5g

Ingredients

1 ½ cups red lentils, soaked overnight and drained

4 ½ cups water

1 sprig rosemary

2 bay leaves

2 roasted peppers, seeded and diced

1 shallot, chopped

2 cloves garlic, minced

1/4 cup olive oil

2 tablespoons tahini

Sea salt and ground black pepper, to taste

Directions

Add the red lentils, water, rosemary and bay leaves to a saucepan and bring to a boil over high heat. Then, turn the heat to a simmer and continue to cook for 20 minutes or until tender.

Place the lentils in a food processor.

Add in the remaining ingredients and process until everything is well incorporated.

Bon appétit!

Wok-Fried Spiced Snow Pea

(Ready in about 10 minutes | Servings 4)

Per serving : Calories: 196; Fat: 8.7g; Carbs: 23g; Protein: 7.3g

Ingredients

2 tablespoons sesame oil

1 onion, chopped

1 carrot, trimmed and chopped

1 teaspoon ginger-garlic paste

1 pound snow peas

Szechuan pepper, to taste

1 teaspoon Sriracha sauce

2 tablespoons soy sauce

1 tablespoon rice vinegar

Directions

Heat the sesame oil in a wok until sizzling. Now, stir-fry the onion and carrot for 2 minutes or until crisp-tender.

Add in the ginger-garlic paste and continue to cook for 30 seconds more.

Add in the snow peas and stir-fry over high heat for about 3 minutes until lightly charred.

Then, stir in the pepper, Sriracha, soy sauce and rice vinegar and stir-fry for 1 minute more. Serve immediately and enjoy!

Quick Everyday Chili

(Ready in about 35 minutes | Servings 5)

Per serving : Calories: 345; Fat: 8.7g; Carbs: 54.5g; Protein: 15.2g

Ingredients

2 tablespoons olive oil

1 large onion, chopped

1 celery with leaves, trimmed and diced

1 carrot, trimmed and diced

1 sweet potato, peeled and diced

3 cloves garlic, minced

1 jalapeno pepper, minced

1 teaspoon cayenne pepper

1 teaspoon coriander seeds

1 teaspoon fennel seeds

1 teaspoon paprika

2 cups stewed tomatoes, crushed

2 tablespoons tomato ketchup

2 teaspoons vegan bouillon granules

1 cup water

1 cup cream of onion soup

2 pounds canned pinto beans, drained

1 lime, sliced

Directions

In a heavy-bottomed pot, heat the olive oil over medium heat. Once hot, sauté the onion, celery, carrot and sweet potato for about 4 minutes.

Sauté the garlic and jalapeno pepper for about 1 minute or so.

Add in the spices, tomatoes, ketchup, vegan bouillon granules, water, cream of onion soup and canned beans. Let it simmer, stirring occasionally, for about 30 minutes or until cooked through.

Serve garnished with the slices of lime. Bon appétit!

Creamed Black-Eyed Pea Salad

(Ready in about 1 hour | Servings 5)

Per serving : Calories: 325; Fat: 8.6g; Carbs: 48.2g; Protein: 17.2g

Ingredients

1 ½ cups black-eyed peas, soaked overnight and drained

4 scallion stalks, sliced

1 carrot, julienned

1 cup green cabbage, shredded

2 bell peppers, seeded and chopped

2 medium tomatoes, diced

1 tablespoon sun-dried tomatoes, chopped

1 teaspoon garlic, minced

1/2 cup vegan mayonnaise

1 tablespoon lime juice

1/4 cup white wine vinegar

Sea salt and ground black pepper, to taste

Directions

Cover the black-eyed peas with water by 2 inches and bring to a gentle boil. Let it boil for about 15 minutes.

Then, turn the heat to a simmer for about 45 minutes. Let it cool completely.

Place the black-eyed peas in a salad bowl. Add in the remaining ingredients and stir to combine well. Bon appétit!

Chickpea Stuffed Avocados

(Ready in about 10 minutes | Servings 4)

Per serving : Calories: 205; Fat: 15.2g; Carbs: 16.8g; Protein: 4.1g

Ingredients

2 avocados, pitted and sliced in half

1/2 lemon, freshly squeezed

4 tablespoons scallions, chopped

1 garlic clove, minced

1 medium tomato, chopped

1 bell pepper, seeded and chopped

1 red chili pepper, seeded and chopped

2 ounces chickpeas, boiled or cabbed, drained

Kosher salt and ground black pepper, to taste

Directions

Place your avocados on a serving platter. Drizzle the lemon juice over each avocado.

In a mixing bowl, gently stir the remaining ingredients for the stuffing until well incorporated.

Fill the avocados with the prepared mixture and serve immediately. Bon appétit!

Black Bean Soup

(Ready in about 1 hour 50 minutes | Servings 4)

Per serving : Calories: 505; Fat: 11.6g; Carbs: 80.3g; Protein: 23.2g

Ingredients

2 cups black beans, soaked overnight and drained

1 thyme sprig

2 tablespoons coconut oil

2 onions, chopped

1 celery rib, chopped

1 carrot, peeled and chopped

1 Italian pepper, seeded and chopped

1 chili pepper, seeded and chopped

4 garlic cloves, pressed or minced

Sea salt and freshly ground black pepper, to taste

1/2 teaspoon ground cumin

1/4 teaspoon ground bay leaf

1/4 teaspoon ground allspice

1/2 teaspoon dried basil

4 cups vegetable broth

1/4 cup fresh cilantro, chopped

2 ounces tortilla chips

Directions

In a soup pot, bring the beans and 6 cups of water to a boil. Once boiling, turn the heat to a simmer. Add in the thyme sprig and let it cook for about 1 hour 30 minutes or until tender.

Meanwhile, in a heavy-bottomed pot, heat the oil over medium-high heat. Now, sauté the onion, celery, carrot and peppers for about 4 minutes until tender.

Then, sauté the garlic for about 1 minute or until fragrant.

Add the sautéed mixture to the cooked beans. Then, add in the salt, black pepper, cumin, ground bay leaf, ground allspice, dried basil and vegetable broth.

Continue to simmer, stirring periodically, for 15 minutes longer or until everything is cooked through.

Garnish with fresh cilantro and tortilla chips. Bon appétit!

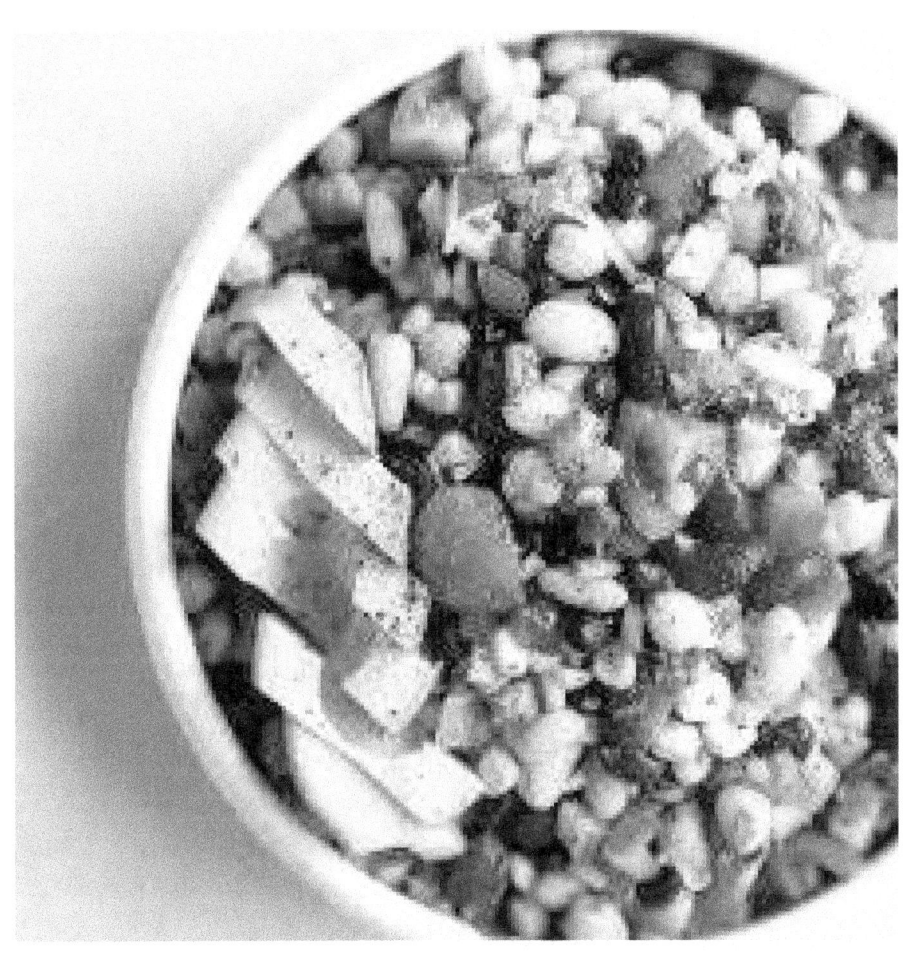

Beluga Lentil Salad with Herbs

(Ready in about 20 minutes + chilling time | Servings 4)

Per serving : Calories: 364; Fat: 17g; Carbs: 40.2g; Protein: 13.3g

Ingredients

1 cup red lentils

3 cups water

1 cup grape tomatoes, halved

1 green bell pepper, seeded and diced

1 red bell pepper, seeded and diced

1 red chili pepper, seeded and diced

1 cucumber, sliced

4 tablespoons shallots, chopped

2 tablespoons fresh parsley, roughly chopped

2 tablespoons fresh cilantro, roughly chopped

2 tablespoons fresh chives, roughly chopped

2 tablespoons fresh basil, roughly chopped

1/4 cup olive oil

1/2 teaspoon cumin seeds

1/2 teaspoon ginger, minced

1/2 teaspoon garlic, minced

1 teaspoon agave syrup

2 tablespoons fresh lemon juice

1 teaspoon lemon zest

Sea salt and ground black pepper, to taste

2 ounces black olives, pitted and halved

Directions

Add the brown lentils and water to a saucepan and bring to a boil over high heat. Then, turn the heat to a simmer and continue to cook for 20 minutes or until tender.

Place the lentils in a salad bowl.

Add in the vegetables and herbs and toss to combine well. In a mixing bowl, whisk the oil, cumin seeds, ginger, garlic, agave syrup, lemon juice, lemon zest, salt and black pepper.

Dress your salad, garnish with olives and serve at room temperature. Bon appétit!

Italian Bean Salad

(Ready in about 1 hour + chilling time | Servings 4)

Per serving : Calories: 495; Fat: 21.1g; Carbs: 58.4g; Protein: 22.1g

Ingredients

3/4 pound cannellini beans, soaked overnight and drained

2 cups cauliflower florets

1 red onion, thinly sliced

1 teaspoon garlic, minced

1/2 teaspoon ginger, minced

1 jalapeno pepper, minced

1 cup grape tomatoes, quartered

1/3 cup extra-virgin olive oil

1 tablespoon lime juice

1 teaspoon Dijon mustard

1/4 cup white vinegar

2 cloves garlic, pressed

1 teaspoon Italian herb mix

Kosher salt and ground black pepper, to season

2 ounces green olives, pitted and sliced

Directions

Cover the soaked beans with a fresh change of cold water and bring to a boil. Let it boil for about 10 minutes. Turn the heat to a simmer and continue to cook for 60 minutes or until tender.

Meanwhile, boil the cauliflower florets for about 6 minutes or until just tender.

Allow your beans and cauliflower to cool completely; then, transfer them to a salad bowl.

Add in the remaining ingredients and toss to combine well. Taste and adjust the seasonings.

Bon appétit!

White Bean Stuffed Tomatoes

(Ready in about 10 minutes | Servings 3)

Per serving : Calories: 245; Fat: 14.9g; Carbs: 24.4g; Protein: 5.1g

Ingredients

3 medium tomatoes, cut a thin slice off the top and remove pulp

1 carrot, grated

1 red onion, chopped

1 garlic clove, peeled

1/2 teaspoon dried basil

1/2 teaspoon dried oregano

1 teaspoon dried rosemary

3 tablespoons olive oil

3 ounces canned white beans, drained

3 ounces sweet corn kernels, thawed

1/2 cup tortilla chips, crushed

Directions

Place your tomatoes on a serving platter.

In a mixing bowl, stir the remaining ingredients for the stuffing until everything is well combined.

Fill the avocados and serve immediately. Bon appétit!

Winter Black-Eyed Pea Soup

(Ready in about 1 hour 5 minutes | Servings 5)

Per serving : Calories: 147; Fat: 6g; Carbs: 13.5g; Protein: 7.5g

Ingredients

2 tablespoons olive oil

1 onion, chopped

1 carrot, chopped

1 parsnip, chopped

1 cup fennel bulbs, chopped

2 cloves garlic, minced

2 cups dried black-eyed peas, soaked overnight

5 cups vegetable broth

Kosher salt and freshly ground black pepper, to season

Directions

In a Dutch oven, heat the olive oil over medium-high heat. Once hot, sauté the onion, carrot, parsnip and fennel for 3 minutes or until just tender.

Add in the garlic and continue to sauté for 30 seconds or until aromatic.

Add in the peas, vegetable broth, salt and black pepper. Continue to cook, partially covered, for 1 hour more or until cooked through.

Bon appétit!

Red Kidney Bean Patties

(Ready in about 15 minutes | Servings 4)

Per serving : Calories: 318; Fat: 15.1g; Carbs: 36.5g; Protein: 10.9g

Ingredients

12 ounces canned or boiled red kidney beans, drained

1/3 cup old-fashioned oats

1/4 cup all-purpose flour

1 teaspoon baking powder

1 small shallot, chopped

2 cloves garlic, minced

Sea salt and ground black pepper, to taste

1 teaspoon paprika

1/2 teaspoon chili powder

1/2 teaspoon ground bay leaf

1/2 teaspoon ground cumin

1 chia egg

4 tablespoon olive oil

Directions

Place the beans in a mixing bowl and mash them with a fork.

Thoroughly combine the beans, oats, flour, baking powder, shallot, garlic, salt, black pepper, paprika, chili powder, ground bay leaf, cumin and chia egg.

Shape the mixture into four patties.

Then, heat the olive oil in a frying pan over a moderately high heat. Fry the patties for about 8 minutes, turning them over once or twice.

Serve with your favorite toppings. Bon appétit!

Homemade Pea Burgers

(Ready in about 15 minutes | Servings 4)

Per serving : Calories: 467; Fat: 19.1g; Carbs: 58.5g; Protein: 15.8g

Ingredients

1 pound green peas, frozen and thawed

1/2 cup chickpea flour

1/2 cup plain flour

1/2 cup breadcrumbs

1 teaspoon baking powder

2 flax eggs

1 teaspoon paprika

1/2 teaspoon dried basil

1/2 teaspoon dried oregano

Sea salt and ground black pepper, to taste

4 tablespoons olive oil

4 hamburger buns

Directions

In a mixing bowl, thoroughly combine the green peas, flour, breadcrumbs, baking powder, flax eggs, paprika, basil, oregano, salt and black pepper.

Shape the mixture into four patties.

Then, heat the olive oil in a frying pan over a moderately high heat. Fry the patties for about 8 minutes, turning them over once or twice.

Serve on burger buns and enjoy!

Black Bean and Spinach Stew

(Ready in about 1 hour 35 minutes | Servings 4)

Per serving : Calories: 459; Fat: 9.1g; Carbs: 72g; Protein: 25.4g

Ingredients

2 cups black beans, soaked overnight and drained

2 tablespoons olive oil

1 onion, peeled, halved

1 jalapeno pepper, sliced

2 peppers, seeded and sliced

1 cup button mushrooms, sliced

2 garlic cloves, chopped

2 cups vegetable broth

1 teaspoon paprika

Kosher salt and ground black pepper, to taste

1 bay leaf

2 cups spinach, torn into pieces

Directions

Cover the soaked beans with a fresh change of cold water and bring to a boil. Let it boil for about 10 minutes. Turn the heat to a simmer and continue to cook for 50 to 55 minutes or until tender.

In a heavy-bottomed pot, heat the olive oil over medium heat. Once hot, sauté the onion and peppers for about 3 minutes.

Sauté the garlic and mushrooms for approximately 3 minutes or until the mushrooms release the liquid and the garlic is fragrant.

Add in the vegetable broth, paprika, salt, black pepper, bay leaf and cooked beans. Let it simmer, stirring periodically, for about 25 minutes or until cooked through.

Afterwards, add in the spinach and let it simmer, covered, for about 5 minutes. Bon appétit!

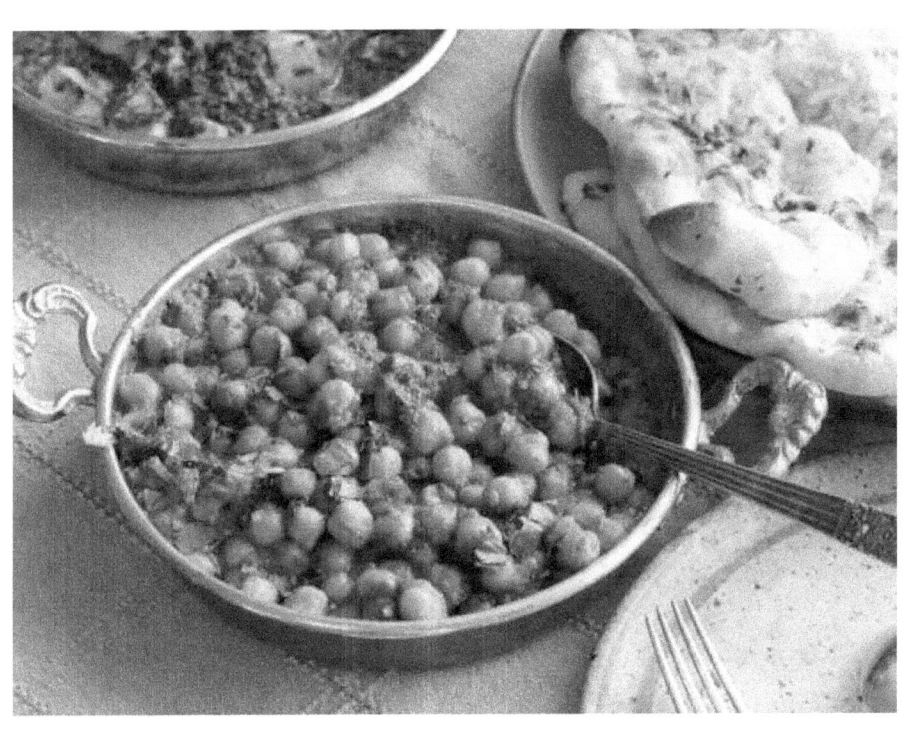

Rainbow Chickpea Salad

(Ready in about 30 minutes | Servings 4)

Per serving : Calories: 378; Fat: 24g; Carbs: 34.2g; Protein: 10.1g

Ingredients

16 ounces canned chickpeas, drained

1 medium avocado, sliced

1 bell pepper, seeded and sliced

1 large tomato, sliced

2 cucumber, diced

1 red onion, sliced

1/2 teaspoon garlic, minced

1/4 cup fresh parsley, chopped

1/4 cup olive oil

2 tablespoons apple cider vinegar

1/2 lime, freshly squeezed

Sea salt and ground black pepper, to taste

Directions

Toss all the ingredients in a salad bowl.

Place the salad in your refrigerator for about 1 hour before serving.

Bon appétit!

Mediterranean-Style Lentil Salad

(Ready in about 20 minutes + chilling time | Servings 5)

Per serving : Calories: 348; Fat: 15g; Carbs: 41.6g; Protein: 15.8g

Ingredients

1 ½ cups red lentil, rinsed

1 teaspoon deli mustard

1/2 lemon, freshly squeezed

2 tablespoons tamari sauce

2 scallion stalks, chopped

1/4 cup extra-virgin olive oil

2 garlic cloves, minced

1 cup butterhead lettuce, torn into pieces

2 tablespoons fresh parsley, chopped

2 tablespoons fresh cilantro, chopped

1 teaspoon fresh basil

1 teaspoon fresh oregano

1 ½ cups cherry tomatoes, halved

3 ounces Kalamata olives, pitted and halved

Directions

In a large-sized saucepan, bring 4 ½ cups of the water and the red lentils to a boil.

Immediately turn the heat to a simmer and continue to cook your lentils for about 15 minutes or until tender. Drain and let it cool completely.

Transfer the lentils to a salad bowl; toss the lentils with the remaining ingredients until well combined.

Serve chilled or at room temperature. Bon appétit!

www.ingramcontent.com/pod-product-compliance
Lightning Source LLC
Chambersburg PA
CBHW071818080526
44589CB00012B/843